MW00415736

Written by: Carmella Sebastian, MD, MS.
Edited by: Jill Westfall
Illustrated by: Jordi Sabaté

ISBN-10: 1482384795
ISBN-13: 978-1482384796

Sex and Spaghetti Sauce

My Italian Mother's Recipe for Getting Healthy
and Getting Busy in Your 50s and Beyond

CARMELLA SEBASTIAN MD, MS

"Not only will you find Dr. Carm's book a valued guide to healthy living, you will find her ability to blend humor with real life experiences a must read for a balanced and happy life. As someone who has known Carm for nearly 20 years, I can attest that you'll be learning from not only a physician, but from a woman with a passion for health and a zest for life!"

Denise S. Cesare, FACHE
President & Chief Executive Officer, Blue Cross of Northeastern Pennsylvania

"If you believe the information overload of health advice and conflicting overdose of dieting info is tripping up millions of us - and I do - than Dr. Carm's book is a simple, straight forward and REALISTIC approach to living happy, health lives with tons of vitality. Oh...and this is one funny lady, too!"

Gary Marino,
Author of *Big & Tall Chronicles: Misadventures of a Lifelong Food Addict!*
Producer & Star - "Million Calorie March: The Movie"

"Sex and spaghetti Sauce: My Italian Mother's Recipe for Getting Healthy and Getting Busy in your 50s and Beyond is an excellent contribution to the health education and health promotion literature. It also represents a very easy and fun read. Dr. Sebastian brings years of wellness experience to the field of learning about healthy living. I highly recommend this very interesting book to anyone who is interested in learning a few things they didn't know about health and happiness as they learn what they thought they already knew."

Bernard J Healey Ph. D.,
Professor of Health Care Administration, King's College, Wilkes-Barre, Pennsylvania
Author of Foundations of Health Care Management, Introduction to Occupational Health in Public Health Practice, Transforming Public Health Practice, and The New World of Health Promotion

To mom and dad. What more can I say?

To Louis and my girls, Gabby and Angie, thank you for your support and unconditional love.

CONTENTS

1

The Family

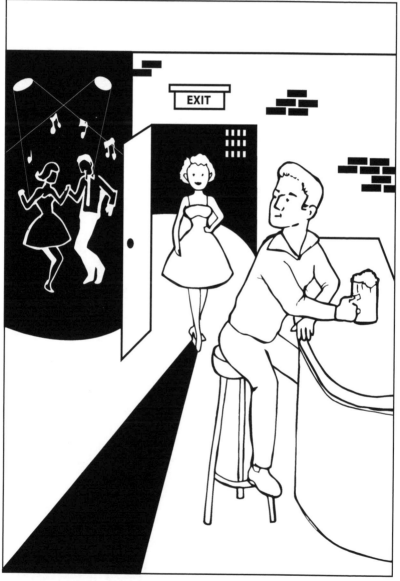

M ary Catanzariti was a gorgeous young woman who walked into a neighborhood bar in Plains, Pennsylvania in 1955. About five feet two inches tall, she had jet-black hair and a 40D bosom. Bosom is what they called "the girls" in the 1950s. Wearing a low-cut, white dress, she was stunning. She was with her best friend, Arlene, and they'd just ditched their dates for the night. As Mary approached the bar, a very handsome man said, "Hi, doll."

That was the start of it all.

His name was Jimmy Mitchell (Americanized from Miceli). He was five feet eleven inches tall with black hair, a Roman nose and a muscular build. Their conversation began with a confession. She told him she was "out on her boyfriend." This meant that she was cheating. He admitted that his girlfriend had no idea where he was that night. They danced, talked, dated, got engaged, were married, and stayed together for 51 years, "till death did them part", just the way it's supposed to happen. The product of this union was one child, me.

Our house was not always peaceful. My parents could fight, and fight good. But, there was laughter with the tears, hugs with the screaming, and food. Really, really good food, all the time. I think they coined the phrase "food is love."

They loved me right into childhood obesity.

In fourth grade, I was four feet tall and weighed 140 pounds. That's obese. It hurt. It hurt when my mom and I went to buy my first pair of bikini underpants and the saleslady tried to sell us "granny panties." It hurt when kids made fun of me. My self-confidence was nil.

But then, a strange thing happened. I started to like boys. These boys liked skinny girls. I also got my period. Somehow I lost all the weight.

I noticed that underneath all that blubber was a nice little body. Other people noticed it, too. Through two pregnancies and a 45-pound weight gain with each, I have been able to stay healthy and fit.

Neither Mary nor Jim ever finished high school. So when I was accepted into medical school, the extended family was all abuzz. I swear that my father could say doctor in five different Italian dialects. He wanted to make sure that everyone understood that his daughter was going to medical school. My mother, on the other hand, could not bear my being two hours away in Philadelphia. So she promptly threw herself on the bed, put a cold towel on her head and cried for a week. She recovered some years later when I bought her a house and gave her two beautiful granddaughters. I was forgiven for leaving her.

My formal education was really wonderful. I attended medical school at the Medical College of Pennsylvania. It was known for being the first women's medical school in the United States (thank God they went co-ed a decade before I got there). I did my internal medicine residency at the Scranton-Temple Residency Program in Scranton, Pa. It was a terrific program near my hometown of Pittston, Pa.

But as wonderful as my formal education was, I learned as much, if not more, from my parents.

I do not want to suggest that they did everything

correctly. What parent does? I have certainly not been a perfect parent. Just ask my 19-year-old daughter! However, they knew more about healing the mind and body than many medical professionals. They used olive oil to cure cradle cap, honey to heal a sore throat, and Epsom salts to relax sore muscles. They drank red wine for longevity, exfoliated with lemon for glowing skin, and practiced deep breathing to maximize balance (and minimize arguments). My parents made health and wellness a lifestyle.

There were some oddities.

Early in life, my father took to curing my migraines by following an age-old superstition called the "malocchio," or evil eye. According to the belief, my headaches were a sign that I'd been "cursed" by someone's envy towards me.

Following the ritual, my dad would sit by my bed and make the sign of the cross on my forehead and whisper some words. If he then sneezed three times, I had, in fact, been cursed and the curse was removed. If not, it was just a headache and an aspirin would do. I can remember only twice when he did not sneeze. I was obviously a very cursed kid. It was probably my new skinny body.

Everyone wanted me!

Along with the malocchio, I learned some very useful information about diet, exercise, love, life, and yes, even sex. As I am now in my early 50s, everything they told me makes perfect sense. Well, in a strange, twisted way, perhaps. But in general, they kept it simple, lived a Mediterranean lifestyle, surrounded themselves with like-minded people, and stayed happy and healthy well into their 80s.

As life grows more and more complex, we all need that common sense wisdom today more than ever. In the next few chapters, I'd like to share with you their wisdom, and I promise you that by incorporating a few of these gems into your everyday life, you will live longer, laugh often, and be a healthier person.

Moderation

or

"I was so depressed that you were a skinny baby, I fed you milkshakes..."

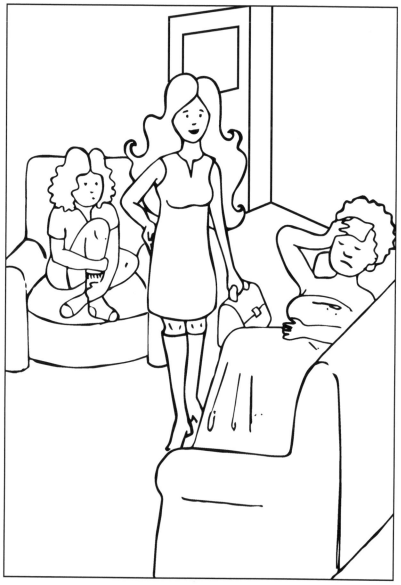

As I said, I was an obese child. I often wondered how I got that way. One day, after the fat was gone, my mother and I were looking through a photo album. There I was as a baby, completely naked. Funny thing is, I was skinny. Not "kid with malnutrition" skinny, but very thin.

I said, "Look at me. I was a thin baby! What happened?"

Mom said, "Oh, I was so upset with you being skinny. I thought you looked sick so I fed you 'till you looked healthy."

"You mean the fat was on purpose?"

"Oh, yes," she answered. "It's amazing how much weight you put on with those milkshakes every night!"

Clearly, other children were not loved as much

as I was since they were not getting nightly milk-shakes.

Let's just say that childhood obesity set me apart, and not in a good way. Unfortunately, I would have a lot of company today. According to the Centers for Disease Control (CDC), the "percentage of children aged 6–11 years in the United States who were obese increased from seven percent in 1980 to nearly 20 percent in 2008. Similarly, the percentage of adolescents aged 12–19 years who were obese increased from five percent to 18 percent over the same period."

That means that almost one in five youth between the ages of six and 19 is obese. Obesity is defined as a body mass index (BMI) of greater than, or equal to, the 95th percentile of the CDC growth chart.

Most of these obese children become overweight, unhealthy adults. Obesity has become a major health concern. One in every three adults is obese; 61.8 percent of women over 20 years of age are overweight and 33 percent of these women are obese. Adults who are obese (a body mass index ≥ 30) have a 50 to 100 percent greater risk of premature death from all causes than people who are at a healthy weight.

Furthermore, premature death results from the progression of chronic illness, and many chronic illnesses are caused or exacerbated by obesity.

In a recent study by RAND Corporation (a global, nonprofit think tank), 133 million Americans – almost one out of every two adults – has at least one chronic illness. According to the CDC, seven out of 10 deaths among Americans each year are from chronic diseases. Heart disease, cancer and stroke account for more than 50 percent of all deaths each year.

In addition, chronic illnesses lead to major disabilities and diminished quality of life. Examples include arthritis, stroke and blindness from diabetes. More than 60 percent of leg and foot amputations, unrelated to injury, are the result of diabetes. One particularly disabling condition related to chronic illness is depression. Almost everyone diagnosed with a chronic medical illness battles depression at some point during the course of their disease.

The connection between obesity and chronic illnesses – like diabetes, high blood pressure, heart disease and arthritis – has long been established.

Only in the past 20 years has the connection been made to cancer. We now understand that obesity is a risk factor for cancers such as uterine, breast and colon, to name a few.

What causes obesity and how did we get here? Genetics, diet, and a sedentary lifestyle all contribute to the increase in childhood obesity. However, being overweight is generally the result of a mismatch between "calories IN" and "calories OUT." Unless you have an underlying problem, like hypothyroidism, you either eat too much, exercise too little, or both.

We know that "calories in" has been affected to a large degree by the fast-food craze of the last few decades and our desire to have bigger and bigger portion sizes. Most of us do not know what a normal portion size looks like anymore. Also, "calories out" has declined with more Americans using cars rather than walking or biking. And never mind all the fantastic technology that allows us to sit on our ever-expanding butts while we watch TV, play video games, and engage in social networking.

Healthy Eating

As in most Italian households, food was a critical aspect of our family's culture. Every celebration, bereavement and holiday was a reason to enjoy great food. I often wondered how Mom and Dad stayed healthy and active into their late 80s. They were never "skinny." But they lived simply and healthfully.

As a young adult, I reflected on how and what we ate. In so doing, I learned the cornerstones of healthy eating within the Miceli household, which is supported by medicine. First, moderation is critical.

Moderation would not be a word that I immediately associate with my mother. However, she did exhibit moderation in many areas of her life. Most importantly were the ones that dealt with health and wellness.

Portion Control or *"Dr. Beratini prescribes dessert ..."*

It's no wonder that I became a doctor. My mother had a fascination with and true appreciation for physicians. My first memory of my mother's physician was when I was around the age of eight and Mom was 48. She was having a hard time with the "change of life," as it was called in those days. She was lying on the couch with a cold towel on her head (again!) and moaning about one symptom or the other when the doorbell rang. In walked a very young woman.

"Who is this?" I remember saying to myself. "She's a doctor?!"

First of all, it was the early 1970s and this was Northeastern Pennsylvania. You just did not see a female physician every day. She was very pretty and had long black hair down to the middle of her back. The most amazing thing was what she was wearing: white go-go boots. Just like Nancy Sinatra. Our doctor was wearing white go-go boots. I thought I would die! Dr. Diorio was pretty, smart AND fashionable! No doubt, this shaped my belief that physicians were the coolest!

To promote the concept even further, every night at dinner my mother would say the same sentence referencing another doctor after we finished eating.

"Dr. Beratini always said that a little dessert after your meal was good for digestion."

Growing up, I loved this mystery man even though I still have no idea who Dr. Beratini was or if he ever really existed. But apparently "he" believed we didn't need things like yogurt with live cultures to digest our food. We could just eat CAKE! Not tons, mind you. Just enough to help the digestion (wink, wink).

Let's discuss the lesson in all of this. Actually, there are two:

1. Footwear is extremely important and can change your life!

2. You can have your cake and eat it too, as long as you understand portion control.

Portion sizes today are much larger than they were in the past, which means we're taking in far more calories than we realize. Understanding healthy and correct portion sizes is critical to long-term weight management.

Use your hand:

1. Your thumb = one ounce of cheese

2. Tip of your thumb = a teaspoon of margarine

3. A handful = one ounce of nuts, candies or pretzels

4. A man's fist = one cup

5. A woman's fist = a serving of starch, like rice or potatoes

6. A woman's palm = three ounces of meat or poultry

7. A woman's hand (fingers together) = a serving of non-starchy vegetables, like lettuce or broccoli

I like using the hand because you always have it with you. Portion size plates are also available and resemble those plastic plates you see at barbecues. Or you can make your own. First, divide the plate in half. One half is where your vegetables should go. Again, non-starchy vegetables like lettuce, cucumbers and broccoli. The remaining half gets divided into two parts. One part is for your protein (fish, chicken, beef) and the second part is for your starch (rice, potatoes, pasta).

There are also very pretty plates available that have flowers painted on them that represent the three areas. They have a large flower for the vegetable and two smaller flowers for the protein and the starch. Check out Slimware plates at **www.fabulousfoods.com.**

Dr. Carm's Recipe for Portion Control:

- Aim for at least half of your plate to be filled with fresh vegetables. Or use a serving size equivalent to the size of your hand (fingers and all).

- Add protein (lean protein is best) to one-half of the remaining area of the plate, or use the palm of your hand as a guide.

- Add starch to the remainder of the plate, which should be about the size of your fist.

- Go easy on fats like butter and margarine and remember your thumb!

- Don't deprive yourself of dessert.

Add half of a cup of ice cream (your fist), a small cookie or a piece of cake (no bigger than your palm) on occasion.

You Can Eat Meat or *"If you want to drive your daughter crazy, order a BLT ..."*

My mother really bought into the "pork fat is good" mentality. She loved bacon. But it had to be well done, and she would order her BLT like this:

"I'd like a plate and on the plate, I'd like two strips of bacon, well done and no extra grease on the grill. I'd like some rye toast, dry, and no butter. I have an allergy to butter. Also, two slices of tomato."

Me: "Mom, why don't you just get a BLT?"

Mom: "No, I have to have it just like that."

Now this forced me to do two things:

1. Tip the server 40 percent, because who in their right mind wouldn't spit in the food of this crazy lady?

2. Sneak butter into the dish every time I made

her a BLT. I knew she did not really have an allergy to butter, so I would sit and watch her eat the sandwich and just smile to myself as she ate every bite. After all, cow fat is good too.

Let's talk about fat.

There are three nutrients that make up our food and they are proteins (think meats, fish and beans), carbohydrates (think fruits and pasta), and fats (butter and oil are examples). Fats are a source of stored energy for our bodies and this is supplied in the form of calories. Fats have more than twice as many calories per gram (nine calories) than proteins or carbohydrates (four calories per gram in each of these). All fats are combinations of saturated and unsaturated fatty acids.

Fatty acids are not produced by the body, so we need to get them from food. They help us with blood clotting, brain function, maintaining healthy skin and hair, and controlling inflammation. Fat is stored in adipose cells, which insulate the body and supply energy. But in excess, fat causes heart disease, cancer and extreme stress during bathing suit season.

Saturated fats are the biggest cause of high LDL

(low-density lipoprotein or "bad cholesterol"). The amount of saturated fat in foods can be found on food labels. Avoid any foods that are high in saturated fats. Saturated fats are found in butter, cheese, whole milk, ice cream, and fatty meats, and can cause heart disease and some forms of cancer.

Unsaturated fats are low in cholesterol, but they still have quite a few calories, so limit them. Some examples include olive oil, canola oil, fish oil, and sunflower oil.

Trans-fatty acids are found in processed foods like cookies, donuts, and some margarines. They are a major contributor to heart disease as they raise the bad cholesterol (LDL) and lower the "good cholesterol" (high-density lipoprotein, or HDL).

Dr. Carm's Recipe for Eating Meat, Oil and Fats:

- Choose lean, protein-rich foods such as soy, fish, skinless chicken, very lean beef, and fat-free or one percent dairy products.

- Limit fried foods, processed foods, and

commercially prepared baked goods
(donuts, cookies, crackers).

- Limit animal products such as egg yolks,
  cheeses, whole milk, cream, ice cream,
  and fatty meats (and large portions of
  beef).

- Look on food labels for words like
  "hydrogenated" or "partially
  hydrogenated," since these foods are
  loaded with bad fats and should be
  avoided.

- Olive and other mono-saturated fat
  oils, soft margarine, and trans fat free
  margarine are preferable to butter, stick
  margarine or shortening.

- Children under the age of two should
  NOT be on a fat-restricted diet because
  cholesterol and fat are thought to be
  important nutrients for brain
  development.

- It is important to read nutrition labels
  and be aware of the amount of different
  types of fat contained in food. If you are

20 or older, ask your healthcare provider about your cholesterol levels.

Dairy is a Girl's Best Friend or *"Hap a cup of coffee with real homo milk ..."*

My mother never ordered a cup of coffee without letting the server know that:

1. She only wanted the cup filled halfway (pronounced "hap") with coffee.

2. She wanted real milk (i.e., not cream) to fill the rest of the cup.

The "homo" part has nothing to do with the sexual preference of the cow. She meant that she wanted homogenized milk in which the milk and cream were mixed together. This was not always available when she was growing up.

My mother's behavior accomplished three things. First, it solidified our position as the least desirable customers in the local restaurants. Second, it ensured that my mother probably never had more than 10 ounces of coffee a day. Third, and most importantly, my mother got her recommended daily allowance of dairy calcium each day.

Dairy calcium has been shown to be an excellent way to accelerate weight loss. A study published in 2003 in the American Journal of Clinical Nutrition involved placing 32 obese patients on a lower-calorie diet. The participants were divided into three groups: a standard control group that received 400 to 500 mg of dietary calcium daily, a high-calcium group that received an 800 mg calcium supplement daily, and a high-dairy group that received 1,200 to 1,300 mg of dietary calcium daily.

What did the study reveal?

It showed that women consuming high dairy calcium are less likely to be obese than women consuming little dairy calcium or even supplemental calcium. The percent of body weight lost and the percent of abdominal fat loss on the low-calorie diet was highest in the dairy group.

And while Mom was staying trim by consuming dairy products, she was also strengthening her bones. Women today have significant issues meeting the recommended daily amount of calcium to protect their bones. As a result, osteoporosis and low bone mass are major public health threats for approximately 55 percent of the U.S. population, 50 years of age and older. Eighty percent (or 35 million individuals) of those affected by osteoporosis are women. Roughly four in 10 white women age 50 or older in the United States will experience a hip, spine, or wrist fracture sometime during their lives.

The number of hip fractures could double or triple by 2020 because of the aging of our population.

How much calcium do we need? The current recommendation is 1,000 to 1,300 mg per day. Foods that are rich in calcium include low-fat milk (an eight-ounce glass has 300 mg of calcium), calcium-fortified orange juice (an eight-ounce glass has 300 mg), an ounce of cheese (which has anywhere from 100 to 250 mg depending on the type of cheese) and broccoli (a half cup has 89 mg of calcium). Check out WebMD. They have a great article on dietary calcium.

Vitamin D is another important component of bone health. Studies have found that low levels have been linked to breast cancer, colon cancer, ovarian cancer, high blood pressure and stroke. Historically, we were told to get our vitamin D from sun exposure. However, if we are protecting ourselves from the harmful rays of the sun by using sunscreen, we will not absorb enough.

Vitamin D is abundant in cooked salmon (3 1/2 ounces has 400 IU), tuna (three ounces has 200 IU) and vitamin D-fortified orange juice and milk (there's approximately 90 IU in one cup). Vitamin D is also contained in many dietary supplements. The preferred supplement form is vitamin D3 since it increases the amount of active vitamin D in our blood and tissues.

How much should we take? The recommended level has been 400 to 600 IU per day, but experts have been lobbying for a new recommended level of 1,000 IU daily for adults (Vieth, 2007). The Food and Nutritional Board at the Institute of Medicine began reviewing the published studies in 2008 and is expected to publish new guidelines.

In the meantime, there's a blood test to determine your level of vitamin D. You can get tested for a baseline level and then test periodically after you start supplementation.

We will speak about exercise later in the book. However, I'd be remiss if I didn't mention the role of weight-bearing exercises in bone health. The current recommendation is for 20 minutes of weight-bearing exercises at least twice per week. You can meet this goal easily by walking with hand weights and doing simple upper-body exercises (like bicep curls or shoulder presses).

Don't smoke. Period. End of discussion. It's the worst thing for every part of your body, including your bones. If you do currently smoke, put down this book, call your doctor, and create a plan to quit. Besides all the over-the-counter aides available, Chantix, a prescription medication, when coupled with behavior modification, has shown impressive results in helping smokers to quit.

In some cases, food allergies, lactose intolerance, or a medical condition like kidney stones may prevent someone from being able to consume dairy or take supplementation. Thankfully, for those who are lactose intolerant, we have lactose-free dairy products. Speak to your physician about a strategy to maintain calcium levels if you have one of these issues. You might also consider trying some of the many nut, seed, or grain milks that are popping up in the dairy case or in shelf-stable cartons in the alternative dairy section of supermarkets and health food stores. Many of these, such as almond, rice, soy and sunflower milks, are fortified with calcium and vitamin D and are excellent choices for people who don't like or cannot tolerate dairy products.

Dr. Carm's Recipe for Bone Health:

- Get adequate calcium (1,000 to 1,500 mg daily). Dietary calcium is best.

- Get adequate vitamin D (400 to 1,000 IU daily).

- Do weight-bearing exercises: aim for 20 minutes, at least two times per week.

- Get or remain smoke-free.

- Obtain regular bone-density tests.

Share at Mealtime or *"Your father is eating all my food!"*

When we ate at home as we did most nights, the portions were small. Although it's clear to me now, I never actually thought about how small Mom's portions were. The rules of filling your plate with protein the size of your palm, carbohydrates the size of your fist, and the rest of the plate with veggies was just how she rolled. I never remember seeing her eat an entire sandwich.

Mom was not super thin, but she ate when she was hungry, stopped when she was full, and that pretty much did the trick for her. She ate slowly and never while sitting in front of the television. Good rules to live by.

As Mom and Dad got older, they started to eat out more. And while my mom never ate everything on her plate, many times the plate was empty when the server came for it. The secret: my dad was eating her food. It was funny because sometimes he would start in on her plate way before she was ready to turn it over. She would just look over at him with an "Are you kidding me?" look.

"Jimmy, do you want to order something else?"

"No," he'd say. "I'll just help you out here."

I am extremely particular when ordering when we go out to eat. My husband and I have developed the following strategy for eating healthy in restaurants:

- Order ice water with lemon. We never order soda and only occasionally a glass of wine, and only after the water. Water hydrates the body and fills you up. Soda provides empty calories with no real nutritional value. More on that later.

- Send the bread basket back as soon as it comes out. Bread will ruin your appetite for the really nutritional food you have coming, and it is usually made with refined flour, not whole grains.

- Avoid ordering appetizers. Think about it. How often do you serve appetizers at home? Never. That is, unless you are having a party. It's just another 500 calories or more that will ruin your appetite for dinner.

- SHARE. The idea is simple. The portion sizes are double what you need. We will usually order a cup of soup each and share a sandwich or an entrée salad. Sometimes, we will order two entrees and split a dessert.

- If we are not sharing, we ask for a takeout container when the food is presented and divide it up before we start to eat.

- Order the salad dressing on the side.

You've got an average of 120 calories
in one tablespoon of most salad dressings.
Try to stick with an olive oil-based
vinaigrette instead of the creamy stuff
and ask for it on the side. This way,
you control how much goes on the salad.

• Don't forget Dr. Beratini and share a
  small piece of pie.

Nutrition Strategies
or
"Buy fresh and don't throw the cauliflower down the toilet."

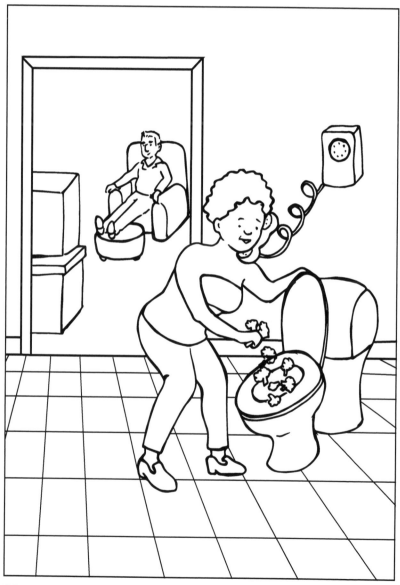

Mom and Dad frequented the local farmers' market, which ran from June through November. Every week my father would take a list from Mom and head to downtown Pittston to take advantage of the local produce. One of Dad's favorite meals was spaghetti with cauliflower. This is a very simple dish and very healthy. It's made with olive oil, garlic and this wonderful cruciferous vegetable. The dish gets big points for helping to fight the development of cancer and for keeping our arteries open.

So one day when I was busy with work and in the car with my boss, I got a call.

Me: "Hi Mom, why are you whispering?"

Mom: "Because I don't want your father to hear."

Me: "What's wrong?"

Mom: "I have a problem. Your father went to the farmers' market and brought home two cauliflowers. They are the size of my head. He got them both for $3."

Me: "So what's the problem?"

Mom: "Well, I don't have time to make two cauli-flowers, so I flushed one down the toilet."

Me: "You mean AFTER you cooked it?"

Mom: "No, raw cauliflower. And now the toilet won't flush!"

Me: "But, Mom, you have a garbage disposal. If you were going to get rid of it, why didn't you put it in the disposal?"

Mom: "Because I didn't want to break the dispos-al. Do you know the phone number for the Ro-to-Rooter man?"

The Benefits of Homegrown

Dad and I planted a garden every year, as did most members of our extended family. We would plant in late April and benefit from the fresh produce all year. First, we would enjoy the fresh produce right out of the ground and then we would can the rest for the winter. We planted onions, garlic, tomatoes, all varieties of squash, root vegetables, lettuces, and cucumbers.

"When you buy locally grown, you're getting the produce at its peak form," says Darlene Price, senior nutrition resource educator at Orange County Cornell Cooperative Extension. "It's ready to eat right now. When you buy your fresh produce in a supermarket, you're never really sure how long it's been sitting."

Much of the produce sold at large supermarket chains is grown hundreds of miles away, in places such as California, Florida, and Mexico. That means that days and perhaps even more than a week have passed since it was picked, packaged, and trucked to the store, where it can sit on the shelves even longer. Often, too, produce is picked before it's ready, preventing it from ever reaching its nutritional potential.

Fruits and vegetables contain essential vitamins, minerals and fiber that may help protect you from many diseases. Most of us aren't consuming enough of them. Studies have shown that those who eat more generous amounts, as part of a healthful diet, are likely to have a reduced risk of chronic diseases, including diabetes, heart disease, and cancer. Fruits and vegetables also contain a high percentage of water and are low in calories. For those of us who are always dealing with trying to lose those "last five pounds," fruits and vegetables should be a major part of our meal plan.

Pick the fruits and vegetables that have vibrant colors. Dark green spinach, orange sweet potatoes, yellow corn, purple plums, and red watermelon all offer excellent health benefits. Spinach and asparagus have large amounts of folate. For potassium, eat tomatoes, potatoes, beets, and drink prune juice.

Speaking of prune juice, my mother had a thing about prunes. Bowel movements were very important to her. Strangely, I hear the same from many of my Italian friends.

My mother raised the prune to food superstar status. She would have prunes in various forms throughout her day. Stewed prunes, prune juice, prune Danish and dried prunes are but a sample. (I actually buried her with two individually wrapped dried prunes, just in case there weren't enough in heaven.)

For vitamin A and C, add carrots, winter squash, cantaloupe, broccoli and, yes, cauliflower. And remember: while fruits and vegetables are naturally nutritious, it's how you store, clean, and prepare them that will determine how nutritious they are when you eat them.

Dr. Carm's Recipe for Eating Your Fruits and Veggies:

- Store produce unwashed, uncut, and loose in crisper drawers in the refrigerator.

- Before serving, wash all fruits and vegetables in clean water – even those that you peel. Wash them as close as you can to consumption.

- Scrub firm produce with a clean produce brush. Dry all produce with a towel to further reduce any possible bacteria.

- Buy local produce whenever possible. Better yet, grow your own.

- Aim for five to seven servings (one serving is the size of your fist) of fruits and vegetables per day.

- Start your day with fruit. Mom added fresh bananas or dried fruit (including prunes) to oatmeal.

- Freeze fresh fruits, such as grapes, blueberries and chunks of bananas, peaches or mango. Then, enjoy them as a refreshing snack or mix them with yogurt, ice and low-fat milk in a blender to make a smoothie.

- Pack a fruit cup, a box of raisins, or a piece of fruit to take with you to work or school.

- Raw vegetables and fruits are very healthy. If you are going to cook them, use as little water as possible to boil. Or better yet, steam them. Do not cook for long to help the food retain as many nutrients as possible.

- Stuff a pita pocket with veggies and sprouts, and drizzle on low-fat salad dressing.

- Toss pasta with cauliflower, sautéed in olive oil and garlic, and top with shredded parmesan cheese. (Thanks, Dad!)

- Sneak in some extra helpings of produce by adding finely chopped vegetables, such as carrots, eggplant, broccoli or cauliflower, to marinara sauce, soups, stews, and chili.

- Roast your vegetables for a deep, rich flavor. Drizzle them with a little olive oil and roast in an oven set to 425 degrees Fahrenheit until tender. You can also place them on the grill. Just brush them with a little olive oil to prevent sticking, and season with some salt and pepper. Try carrots, asparagus, butternut squash, eggplant and broccoli this way - yum!

- Some fruits and veggies will be more nutritious when cooked, such as tomatoes, which develop their lycopene as they cook. Lycopene gives tomatoes their color and is an antioxidant that has been linked to the prevention of cancer and heart disease.

You may shy away from fresh produce after the

health scares that we have had with melons, tomatoes, and spinach over the past few years. But if you follow some basic food-prep rules, you will be safe. Most cases of food-borne illness can be prevented through the proper cooking or processing of food, which kills bacteria. And remember: because bacteria multiply rapidly between 40 and 140 degrees Fahrenheit, try to keep food out of this temperature range.

Other food handling tips:

- Refrigerate foods promptly. If prepared food stands at room temperature for more than two hours, it may not be safe to eat.

- Set your refrigerator to 40 degrees Fahrenheit or lower and your freezer to zero degrees Fahrenheit.

- Cook food to the appropriate internal temperature – 145 degrees Fahrenheit for roasts, steaks, chops of beef, veal and lamb; 160 degrees Fahrenheit for pork, ground veal and ground beef; 165 degrees Fahrenheit for ground poultry; and 180 degrees Fahrenheit for whole poultry. Use a meat thermometer to be sure. Foods are properly cooked only when they are heated long enough and at a high enough temperature to kill the harmful bacteria that can cause illnesses.

- Prevent cross-contamination. Bacteria can spread from one food product to another throughout the kitchen and can get onto cutting boards, knives, sponges and countertops. Keep raw meat, poultry, seafood and their juices away from all ready-to-eat foods.

- Handle food properly. Always wash your hands for at least 20 seconds with warm, soapy water before and after handling raw meat, poultry, fish, shellfish, produce and eggs. Also, wash your hands after using the bathroom, changing diapers, or touching animals.

- Wash utensils and surfaces before and after use with hot, soapy water. Better still, sanitize with diluted bleach – one teaspoon of bleach to one quart of hot water.

- Wash sponges and dish towels weekly in hot water in the washing machine.

- Keep cold food cold and hot food hot.

- Maintain hot cooked food at 140 degrees Fahrenheit or higher.

- Reheat cooked food to at least 165 degrees Fahrenheit.

- Never defrost food on the kitchen counter. Use the refrigerator, cold running water or the microwave oven.

- Never let food marinate at room temperature – refrigerate it.

- Do not pack the refrigerator. Cool air must circulate to keep food safe.

For more information about the prevention of food-borne illnesses, the U.S. Department of Agriculture provides fact sheets on safe-food handling:**http://www.fsis.usda.gov/Fact_Sheets/ Safe_Food_Handling_Fact_Sheets/**

Eat Out Infrequently or *"Is that corn on the cob?"*

Like I said, I'm very particular about what I eat in restaurants and how often I eat out. But, my mother was the queen of picky ordering.

Mom was never crazy about eating out, generally speaking. She had to love the cuisine (Italian) and she liked to know who ran the restaurant and would often wander into the kitchen.

Imagine what happened at a very upscale Chinese restaurant.

My cousins John and Josette were in the clothing business. Every summer there was a clothing show in Atlantic City. We tagged along and John and Josette were always so gracious. One evening they took us to a Chinese restaurant.

Now, Mom usually only ate Mediterranean fare. She avoided fast-food joints like the plague, no doubt adding years to her life. She did eat a couple of things out: pizza, barbecue, shellfish, and yes, bacon. But in general, she never thought the restaurants were clean enough or made the food with the same love and attention to detail as she did.

So, there we were sitting in a Chinese restaurant and the ambiance was wonderful. This was a very upscale restaurant, so the lights were dimmed. Mom was eating... white rice. It's all she would eat and all she would try. In between courses, the server brought out a rather large platter with what looked like six-inch rolls on it.

Mom exclaims, "Thank God, corn on the cob!"

Well, frankly, from my vantage point, it did look like corn on the cob. But when our family members sitting nearest to the platter realized what it was, they all started to laugh. The rolls were warm hand towels.

No, she didn't eat the towel. She also didn't try to hide her dislike of the choice of restaurant.

Later, she found bacon in a deli and was a happy camper.

I eat out with my family just once a week. Studies have shown that there's less salt and fat in home-cooked meals. According to a 2007 article published by *The Journal of the American Medical Association*, 77 percent of the sodium in the U.S. diet comes from restaurant and processed foods. Twelve percent occurs naturally. We add six percent at the table and sprinkle in five percent during cooking.

Dr. Carm's Recipe for Eating Out and Eating Well:

- When eating out, plan ahead. If you're eating alone, ask for a to-go container as soon as the food is served and place half of it in the container for lunch or dinner tomorrow night. If you are eating with someone, share (see Chapter Two).

- Check out the book *Eat This, Not That! Thousands of Simple Food Swaps that Can Save You 10, 20, 30 Pounds--or More,* by David Zinczenko with Matt Goulding.

- Experience mindful eating. There is an awesome book called *Eat What You Love, Love What You Eat* by Dr. Michelle May. She suggests that before you even enter the restaurant, you ask yourself:

-"Am I hungry?"

-"How hungry am I?"

-"What do I want? What do I need? What do I have?"

• Avoid foods that are heavily seasoned. Examples are blackened meats or fish, soups, dips, and appetizers. Don't be afraid to ask for seasoning or sauces on the side.

• Stick to salads with a broiled or baked protein on the top (like salmon, chicken or shrimp) and ask that they aren't over-seasoned. Remember to get the dressing on the side.

Before I order, I look at what I've eaten all day and what nutrients I'm probably missing. If I've had carbohydrates for breakfast and lunch, I may feel the need for protein at dinner. However, just because I'm in a restaurant doesn't mean that I have to eat a full meal or eat at all. I order what

I feel my body needs and only eat until I'm satisfied, not stuffed.

Whole Grains Are Good or *"Time to wake up and drink the prune juice…"*
Imagine that you are a pre-teen and then a teenager. For a solid ten years, you are woken up in the same way:

Your mom bursts into your room yelling, "Time to wake up!"

And in her hand is a four-ounce glass of prune juice. She insists that you drink this even before getting out of bed.

I know. It's a nightmare.

It took me several years to realize that I could say "no thanks" and then several more to stop defecating every time I saw a small glass of dark liquid. But I didn't miss the lesson: you must eat and drink every morning (or whenever you wake up to start your day).

Mom ate breakfast every day of her life; most of the time she ate oatmeal or a whole grain cereal with milk. There were no studies at that time linking breakfast eaters to successful dieting or weight control, but it was common sense. You were asleep for eight hours. Your body was hungry and thirsty. We wouldn't try to drive a car without putting gas in it first, would we? We should not go eight hours at night, or during the day, without fueling our bodies.

Most experts agree that several smaller meals per day is the most beneficial way to fuel our bodies and control weight. It also keeps our blood sugar levels steady. This is not only good for diabetics but helps the rest of us since blood sugar variations wreak havoc with our cortisol levels, and that has been linked to obesity.

Recent studies have also linked breakfast with weight loss. The National Weight Control Registry showed that the majority of people maintaining weight loss eat breakfast. They analyzed the eating habits of 3,000-plus people (2,350 women) who kept at least 30 pounds off for a year. What they found was that 78 percent of these people eat breakfast daily and most of them are choosing a whole-grain cereal.

Since my mother ate oatmeal most days, it's no wonder that high cholesterol was not an issue for her. And she'd add at least a quarter cup of milk to the oatmeal, along with bananas and berries. The banana was important for potassium since she had high blood pressure ever since giving birth. If she said it once, she said it a hundred times, "You know, I was in labor for over a day. I had toxemia. They had to 'take you' (C-section) because you were drowning."

Yeah, you know, the "I almost died giving birth" routine.

The Skinny on Carbs

I was very depressed in the late 80s when there was a backlash on pasta. First, I am a carb-freak and will be until the day I die. Second, I was raised on the traditional spaghetti and meatballs every Sunday after church. No pasta means no life. Thank God there's a way to enjoy it and be healthy.

Consider this:

One study demonstrated the positive role whole grains play in weight management. Women were randomized to a diet with a low amount of whole grain and a high amount of whole grain.

- At baseline, women in the highest intake group weighed less than did women in the lowest intake group.

- Increases in whole grain intake were associated with significantly less weight gain over time.

- Refined grain (think white!) intake was linked to an increased risk of weight gain.

- Women in the highest group of dietary fiber intake had a 49 percent lower risk of major weight gain.

In conclusion, women who consumed more whole grain consistently weighed less than women who consumed less whole grain. Consider data from the USDA's 1994-96 Continuing Survey of Food Intakes by Individuals, Pyramid Servings Data, published in 2004. The study took 4,776 men and 4,475 women and put them on a diet of no whole grains, less than one serving of whole grain per day, one serving, two servings, and three or more servings.

What they found was that women who consumed

zero servings of whole grains a day had a BMI of 26.4 compared to a BMI of 24.2 in women who ate three or more servings. Men who ate zero servings of whole grains a day had a BMI of 26.3 compared to a BMI of 25.7 in men who ate three or more servings a day.

It's important to realize that a drop in BMI of even one point is clinically significant.

Dr. Carm's Recipe for Weight Management Through Diet:

- Eat breakfast (even if it's only a banana) every day.

- Incorporate whole grains (think brown, not white) into your diet. Examples are brown rice, whole-wheat pasta, whole-grain bread (not "enriched"). It must say "whole grain" or "whole wheat."

- NEVER force your children to drink prune juice!

The Mediterranean Diet

"First we make our habits and then our habits make us."

Charles C. Noble

My mother had some habits that were not acceptable to those who lived with her - or probably to society as a whole. One of them involved the local grocery store. My father did 90 percent of the grocery shopping. I was never sure why but I think it had something to do with him NEEDING to get out of the house and away from her every now and then. He would head out with the list she wrote in hand and return home a couple of hours later. Let me just remind you that there were no cell phones at that time.

When he was in the A&P (the store had many different names over the years that this story took place), he would hear the following on the speaker:

"Jimmy Mitchell, please come to the front desk. You have a call."

The poor man would run to the front desk, sure that someone had just died. Nope. Mary forgot to put a quart of milk on the list. To say that this same activity continued weekly over the span of 20 years would be, in itself, unbelievable, but it wasn't just that. The clerks at the front desk tired of waiting for him to come to the phone, so the message became:

"Jimmy, Mary is on the phone. She needs a quart of milk and a dozen eggs."

My poor father couldn't escape to save his life, not even in the local grocery store.

One typical shopping experience found him standing in the dairy aisle just staring at the milk.

A friend passing by said, "Jim, are you ok?"

Dad said to him: "Sam, you know what happiness is?"
Sam: "No, Jim. What is happiness?"

Dad: "It is seeing your wife's picture on the side of a milk carton."

God, I loved that man.

Paging people was a bad habit that my mother

could not shake. Our family's nutrition was a good habit that she could not shake either, and thank God for that.

We couldn't help but eat a diet of vegetables, olive oil, garlic and healthy grains. We were Italian! It was OUR diet. That was OUR food. There were no studies at the time showing that this was the healthiest way to eat. We were just raised that way. Scientists have intensely studied the eating patterns characteristic of the Mediterranean diet for more than half a century. It started shortly after World War II: Ancel Keys and colleagues (including Paul Dudley White, later President Eisenhower's heart doctor) organized the remarkable Seven Countries Study to examine the hypothesis that Mediterranean-eating patterns led to improved health outcomes. This long-running study examined the health of almost thirteen thousand middle-aged men in the United States, Japan, Italy, Greece, the Netherlands, Finland and then-Yugoslavia.

When the data were examined, it was clear that people who ate a diet based on fruits, vegetables, grains, beans, and fish were healthiest. From this conclusion emerged the concept of a "Mediterranean diet" that could promote lifelong good health. In subsequent years, the body of scientific evidence supporting the healthfulness of the traditional Mediterranean diet continued to grow.

What are the main features of the Mediterranean diet?

The typical diet features foods grown all around the Mediterranean Sea, along with lifestyle factors typical of this region.

Grains should be whole grains, such as wheat, oats, rice, rye, barley, and corn. These grains are best consumed in whole, minimally processed forms, because refining and processing can remove many valuable nutrients, including vitamins, minerals, and fiber.

Vegetables are key in all the countries bordering the Mediterranean Sea. Their benefits are amplified because the vegetables are normally cooked or drizzled with olive oil. Raw vegetables are also a healthy vegetable option. In my opinion, one of the BEST veggies is GARLIC... full of flavor and heart-healthy.

Whole Fresh Fruits are ever-present in the Mediterranean. It's important to know that fruit juices tend to have more sugar and less fiber than their whole-fruit counterparts, and no-sugar-added fruit juices provide only some of the same nutritional benefits as whole fruit.

Olives and olive oil are central to the Mediterranean diet. Olives are universally eaten whole, and widely used for cooking and flavoring in the countries that border the Mediterranean Sea. Olive oil is the principal source of dietary fat used for cooking, baking, and dressing salads and vegetables. Extra-virgin olive oil is highest in health-promoting fats, phytonutrients, and other important micronutrients.

Nuts, beans, legumes and seeds are good sources of healthy fats, protein, and fiber. They add flavor and texture to Mediterranean dishes.

Herbs and spices add flavors and aromas to foods, reducing the need to add salt or fat when cooking. They are also rich in a broad range of health-promoting antioxidants, and are used liberally in Mediterranean cuisines.

Cheese and yogurt are eaten regularly in the traditional Mediterranean diet, but in low to moderate amounts. As you've read, the calcium in cheese and yogurt is important for bone and heart health. Low-fat and nonfat dairy products are best.

Fish and shellfish are important sources of healthy protein for Mediterranean populations. Fish such as tuna, herring, sardines and salmon are rich in essential heart-healthy omega-3 fatty acids. Shellfish and crustaceans - including mussels, clams and shrimp - have similar benefits. Fish and shellfish are not battered and fried in Mediterranean countries.

Eggs are a good source of high-quality protein, and can be especially beneficial for individuals who do not eat meat. Eggs are regularly used in baking as well.

Meats are eaten in small portions by Mediterranean people, who prefer lean cuts. Poultry is a good source of lean protein without the high levels of saturated fat found in some cuts of red meat. With ground meats, 90 percent lean/10 percent fat is a good choice.

Wine is consumed regularly but moderately in the Mediterranean, unless discouraged by religious beliefs. "Moderately" means up to one (1) four-ounce glass of wine per day for women and up to two (2) four-ounce glasses for men. Individuals should only drink wine if they are medically able to do so.

Two newer studies confirm these earlier findings. One study tracked more than 2,300 healthy elderly men and women from eleven different European countries for ten years. Those people with eating habits that met at least half of the criteria of a Mediterranean diet suffered at least 25 percent fewer deaths during that period.

In fact, people who ate a mostly Mediterranean diet, exercised moderately, drank little to moderate amounts of alcohol and didn't smoke had 65 percent fewer deaths than those who followed none or only one of these healthy habits.

The other new study involved people with metabolic syndrome, a disorder linked with heart disease risk. The warning signs for this disorder are waistline obesity, low HDL (good) cholesterol, high blood triglycerides (fats), and insulin resistance. Half of the participants in this study were told to follow a Mediterranean-style diet and the other half a traditional low-fat diet. Both groups were asked to increase their exercise.

In time, the Mediterranean group showed reduced markers for inflammation, which is linked to a risk of heart disease and cancer. Markers for blood vessel health also improved for this group. After two years, less than half of the group on the Mediterranean diet still had metabolic syndrome, while almost everyone on the traditional low-fat diet still had it. A recent review of many studies on the Mediterranean diet found that the risk of heart disease can drop from 45 percent to eight percent if people follow this diet.

In addition to reducing the risk of heart disease and cancer, the Mediterranean diet may help control weight as well. In the new study with people afflicted with metabolic syndrome, those on a Mediterranean diet lost more weight than those on a low-fat diet – a total difference of nine pounds in two years. In an earlier study, a group with a Mediterranean-style diet of moderate fat content lost the same amount of weight at first as another group on a low-fat diet, but the Mediterranean group kept the weight off longer. In fact, only one-fifth of the low-fat group could stick to their diet.

Dr. Carm's Recipe for Eating the Mediterranean Way:

- Create a diet with plenty of vegetables, fruits, and whole grains with daily servings of dried beans, nuts or seeds.

- Consume only small amounts of red meat, if you eat it.

- Serve fish regularly.

- Use olive oil as your main source of fat instead of butter or margarine.

- Choose fruit instead of high-fat, high-sugar desserts and bakery products, except for special occasions.

- Drink alcohol in moderation.

To be fair and complete, let's look at other diets that have been popular in the last few years:

Atkins

The Atkins Diet, or Atkins Nutritional Approach, focuses on controlling the levels of insulin in our bodies. This diet limits refined carbohydrates. If we consume large amounts of refined carbohydrates, our insulin levels will rise rapidly, and then fall rapidly. The premise is that rising insulin levels will trigger our bodies to store as much of the energy we eat as possible. It will also make it less likely that our bodies will use stored fat as a source of energy. Most people on the Atkins Diet will consume a higher proportion of proteins than they normally do. This is NOT a low-fat diet.

The Zone

The Zone Diet aims for a nutritional balance of 40 percent carbohydrates, 30 percent fats and 30 percent protein each time we eat. The focus is also on controlling insulin levels, which can result in more successful weight loss and weight control. The Zone Diet encourages the consumption of good quality carbohydrates – unrefined carbohydrates and fats, such as olive oil, avocado, and nuts.

Vegetarian

There are various types of vegetarian diets - lactovegetarian, fruitarian, lacto-ovo vegetarian, living-food vegetarian, ovo-vegetarian, pesco-vegetarian, and semi-vegetarian. The majority of vegetarians are lacto-ovo vegetarians. In other words, they do not eat animal-based foods, except for eggs, dairy and honey.

Several studies over the last few years have shown that vegetarians have a lower body weight, suffer less from diseases and generally have a longer life expectancy than people who eat meat. Check out an excellent video on YouTube called "Forks over Knives." It will completely change your approach to eating meat.

Vegan

Veganism is more of a way of life and a philosophy than a diet. A vegan does not eat anything that is animal-based, including eggs, dairy and honey. Vegans do not generally adopt veganism just for health reasons, but also for environmental and ethical reasons. They believe that modern intensive farming methods damage the environment and are unsustainable in the long term.

Vegans feel that if all of our foods were plant-based, our environment would benefit, animals would suffer less, more food would be produced, and people would generally enjoy better physical and mental health.

Weight Watchers

Weight Watchers focuses on losing weight through diet, exercise and a support network. Weight Watchers Inc. was born in the 1960s when a housewife lost some weight and was concerned that she might put it back on. So, she created a network of like-minded friends to support each other. Today, Weight Watchers is a huge company with branches all over the world. Dieters can join either physically, and attend regular meetings, or go online. In both cases, there is a great deal of support and education available for the dieter.

South Beach

The South Beach Diet was created by a cardiologist, Dr. Arthur Agatston, and a nutritionist, Marie Almon, as a way to help patients improve their blood chemistries and lose weight in order to prevent heart attacks and strokes. It also focuses on the control of insulin levels, and the benefits of unrefined slow carbohydrates versus highly processed fast carbs. Dr. Agatston devised the South Beach Diet during the 1990s because he was disappointed with the low-fat, high-carb diet backed by the American Heart Association at the time. He believed and found that low-fat diets were not effective over the long-term.

What is the data that supports adoption of any of these diets?

In two studies published in the New England Journal of Medicine in 2003 comparing low-fat and low-carbohydrate diets, researchers found that low-carbohydrate diets produced greater weight loss at six months. But at the one-year mark, weight loss was similar with both diets. The differences in weight loss on a low-carbohydrate diet, versus a low-fat diet, at 12 months were not significant.

Another study in JAMA compared four diets: Atkins, Ornish, Weight Watchers, and the Zone. Researchers found that each diet modestly reduced weight and cardiac risk factors at one year with no significant differences between diets. Researchers found that overall dietary adherence rates, for all the diets, were low.

You want the SECRET to making any of these food plans work for you? Regardless of the "diet" or food regimen that you choose, the real secret is to make habitual changes. Adopting a healthy way of life isn't really healthy unless you can incorporate those habits into your life every day for the rest of your life.

The Mediterranean diet was our habit. I assert that if you can learn an unhealthy, bad habit, you can unlearn it and replace it with a good or better habit.

How can we do this? Let's use what I call the "Six-Step Habit Changer."

Step #1: Ask yourself if you are ready to change.

If you're not sure you want to change, then it's probably not time. Your chances of being successful will be greatly diminished.

This philosophy, and the data to support it, comes from the Prochaska and DiClemente Stages of Change Model. It was originally identified and developed during a study of smoking cessation in 1983. It was then applied and studied with numerous bio-psycho-social problems. I believe that it fits very well with all wellness habits. There are five stages: pre-contemplation, contemplation, preparation, action and maintenance, and relapse prevention.

Pre-contemplation Stage

During the pre-contemplation stage, people do not even consider changing. Smokers who are in denial may not see that the advice applies to them personally. People with high cholesterol levels may feel immune to the health problems that strike others. Obese individuals may have tried unsuccessfully to lose weight so many times that they have simply given up.

Contemplation Stage

During the contemplation stage, people are ambivalent about changing. Giving up an enjoyed behavior causes them to feel a sense of loss despite the perceived gain. During this stage, we assess barriers (e.g.: time, expense, hassle, fear, "I know I need to, doc, but...") as well as the benefits of change.

Preparation Stage

During the preparation stage, people prepare to make a specific change. They may experiment with small changes as their determination to change increases. For example, sampling low-fat foods may be an experiment with , or a move toward, greater dietary modification. Switching to a different brand of cigarettes, or decreasing drinking, signals that they have decided a change is needed.

Action Stage

The action stage is the one that signals a true change is coming. While any action should be praised because it demonstrates true desire for change, failed New Year's resolutions provide evidence that if the prior stages have been glossed over, action itself is often not enough.

Maintenance and Relapse Prevention

Maintenance and relapse prevention entail incorporating the new behavior over the long haul. Discouragement over occasional slips can halt the change process, and most people will find themselves recycling through the stages of change several times before the change becomes truly established.

Okay, so let's say you're ready for true change.

Step #2: Set a goal. A goal for losing weight should not be "wearing a sexy dress to my high school reunion." Unless you are going to wear this dress every day for the rest of your life, this goal does not have staying power.

What do you care about? Getting and staying healthy for your family? Getting off medication? Climbing steps without the need for a respirator? My goal, and reason for wanting to change, is rather simple: I want to take my grandchildren to Disney World (in the far off future, as my two girls are teenagers!) and not have to ride in a scooter. I want to be heard yelling, "Come on now kids, keep up with Grandma!"

Step #3: Make a plan. You MUST write it down. Why does it seem that even when we know that lies can be written down as easily as they are spoken, we still believe the written word over the spoken one? Well, I'm not sure, but let's use it to our advantage. Write down what you honestly need to change to reach your goal. When you are doing this, you will want to do what we do in the business world.

In business we use SMART goals. SMART goals require that we document them. SMART stands for specific, measurable, attainable, realistic and timely.

S = Specific:

In order to be an active senior one day and not have to use a scooter, I need to:

- Exercise for 45 minutes or more, most days of the week, combining cardio and weight training.

- Eat approximately 1,200 to 1,500 calories a day of a diet consisting mostly of whole grains, fruits, and veggies.

- Drink 64 ounces of water each day.

- Know my body and get regular check-ups and appropriate screenings.

You get the idea.

M = Measurable:

- Exercise for 45 minutes is measurable; just "exercise" is not.

- Eating good food is not measurable. Eating approximately 1,200 to 1,500 calories a day of a diet consisting mostly of whole grains, fruits and veggies is measurable.

A = Attainable:

My goal is not to look like Angelina Jolie. I am not going to have Jennifer Aniston's body. NOT EVER. What I do want, which I believe is definitely attainable, is to be the best Carmella I can be. This is what I call your "Wellness Potential."

If you're having difficulty determining whether or not your goal is really possible, or simply a pipe dream, ask a true friend. If you do not have a true friend, forget getting healthy. Find a true friend first.

I hope I've been a true friend. God knows I'm honest. I've tried to only offer advice when asked. But when asked, I give it to you straight.

R = Realistic:

This is important. What happens when we go to Weight Watchers? They weigh us and then they help us determine the goal. They never say, "You are 50 pounds overweight; you need to lose it all in six weeks." The goal is 10 percent of your current weight, or less, depending on your height (essentially, taking your BMI into account). This is realistic and doable.

T = Timely:

You need to assign a time limit to the goal. It can't be "whenever" or "tomorrow." Exercising 45 minutes most days of the week means just that. If you don't feel comfortable with "most days of the week," pick a number. Exercise 45 minutes every day, at least four days a week. Now there's no confusion.

Now, don't give me that look.

You know, the one that says, "I don't have time for this."

Do you have time to do financial planning? Do you have time to plan for your child's college education or wedding? Well, isn't your health at least AS important as that? Don't short change yourself. You need a goal and you need to write it down.

Step #4: Share this plan with someone who cares about you and wants to see you succeed. Why? So they can be there to encourage you and cheer when you have a great day. But most importantly, they can be there to boost you up and help you stay on track when you have a bad day. There will be bad days. That is life.

Step #5: Monitor your progress. Again, by writing it down we will be honest with ourselves and have a record. You do not have to do this forever. But to get you moving in the right direction, I suggest it for at least the first three months. After that, you can use the way your underwear fits, or your measured weight, as evidence of your progress. But you need to have some objective measure. Studies have shown that people who weigh themselves weekly are more successful in keeping the weight off.

Step #6: Repeat and refine as needed.
Make any necessary changes and keep going. Remember that you will relapse and that is okay. Why did you slip-up? How can you avoid that trap next time?

Writing down your goal and what you are honestly doing and checking in with someone who cares about you will allow you to be mindful of what is not working.

Example: "I was exercising 45 minutes, six days a week and I felt exhausted. I was not able to do my best on that sixth day and was just going through the motions. I can handle five days without the associated guilt and still reach my goal."

Perfect, do it! And then do it again, and again... Oh my God, that is the definition of a habit. You keep doing it, over and over, without even thinking about it. Congratulations!

Dr. Carm's Recipe for Habit Change that Sticks:

Step 1: Are you ready to change?

Step 2: Develop a goal.

Step 3: Document your plan and use the "SMART goal" system.

Step 4: Share your plan with someone who cares about you and wants to see you succeed.

Step 5: Monitor your progress.

Step 6: Make changes, relapse, but keep moving forward.

4

Exercise Is the Key
or
"Why should I exercise, I clean the house?"

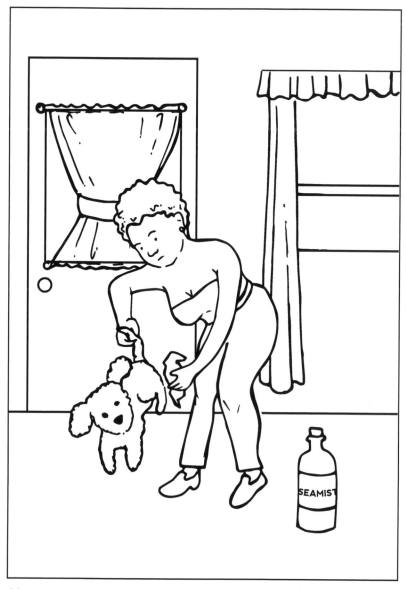

My mother was a clean freak. She would rather receive a compliment on the cleanliness of her house than on what she looked like. She would tell this story proudly.

"A delivery person came to the kitchen door, and he said, "Wow, you could eat off those floors.""

That would make her practically giddy.

The truth is that you COULD eat off of her floors. We had a dog, a poodle named Pierre. She'd wipe that dog's ass with Seamist every time he went out to poop. Those floors never saw a speck of poodle poop. Seamist was a popular brand of ammonia. Pierre lived to be 18 human years old. Everyone said that the ammonia was responsible for his longevity since it probably penetrated his anal area and kept him alive.

When I would suggest that we go for a walk, or get some physical activity, Mom would insist that she did not need to exercise since she cleaned EVERY

DAY. Mom's exercise of choice was cleaning the house.

I decided to test her method and strapped on my heart rate monitor and cleaned my own house. I did not do what Mom would call "heavy" cleaning. I did not move furniture. I dusted, stripped the beds, cleaned the bathrooms and ran the sweeper. I was shocked to see that I had burned almost 200 calories an hour. Damn, she was right again.

This made me realize that the most important part of exercise is just moving. You need to keep moving every day.

Studies have long established that physical activity has beneficial effects on numerous age-related conditions such as osteoarthritis, falls, hip fractures, cardiovascular disease, respiratory diseases, cancer, diabetes mellitus, osteoporosis, low fitness, obesity, and decreased functional capacity.

One of the new studies adds mental deterioration and says that exercise produces "a significantly reduced risk of cognitive impairment after two years for participants with moderate or high physical activity" who were older than 55 when the study began.

Most early studies, demonstrating the benefits of exercise, were done on men. Now many recent studies have shown that active women reap comparable rewards. Skeptics are fond of saying that it is no coincidence that exercise is associated with good health as one ages; the people who exercise are healthy to begin with. But that's simply not true. In one study, some participants were randomly assigned to a physical-activity program and others were just told to exercise. The findings of exercise leading to better health in aging persisted.

In the Nurses' Health Study, Dr. Qi Sun of the Harvard School of Public Health reported that among the 13,535 nurses who were healthy when they joined the study in 1986, those who reported higher levels of activity in midlife were far more likely to still be healthy a decade or more later, at age 70. He and his co-authors found that physical activity increased the nurses' chances of remaining healthy regardless of body weight, although those who were both lean and active had "the highest odds of successful survival."

Reviewing the benefits of exercise one at a time, here are what recent studies have shown, including several studies published in The Archives of

Internal Medicine:

Cancer

In a review last year of 52 studies on exercise and colon cancer, researchers at Washington University School of Medicine in St. Louis concluded that people who were most active were 21 percent less likely to develop cancer than those who were least active, possibly because activity helps to move waste more quickly through the bowel.

The risk of breast cancer, too, is about 16 percent lower among physically active women, perhaps because exercise reduces tissue exposure to insulin-like growth factor, a known cancer promoter.

Indirectly, exercise may protect postmenopausal women against cancers of the endometrium, pancreas, colon, and esophagus, as well as breast cancer, by helping them keep their weight down.

Osteoporosis and fragility

Weak bones and muscles increase the risk of falls and fractures and an inability to perform the tasks of daily life. Weight-bearing aerobic activities like brisk walking, and weight training to increase muscle strength, can reduce, or even reverse bone loss. German researchers who randomly assigned women 65 and older to either an 18-month exercise regimen, or a wellness program, demonstrated that exercise significantly increased bone density and reduced the risk of falls. And, at any age, even in people over 100, weight training improves the size and quality of muscles, thus increasing the ability to function independently.

Cardiovascular disease

Aerobic exercise has long been established as an invaluable protector of the heart and blood vessels. It increases the heart's ability to work hard, lowers blood pressure and raises blood levels of HDL-cholesterol, which act as a cleansing agent in arteries. As a result, active individuals of all ages have lower rates of heart attacks and strokes.

A 2002 study was published in The New England Journal of Medicine by Dr. JoAnn E. Manson and colleagues. The study found that among 73,743 initially healthy women, ages 50 to 79 who walked briskly for 30 minutes a day, five days a week, there was a substantial reduction in the risk of heart attacks and other cardiovascular events.

In another study, women who walked at least one hour a day were 40 percent less likely to suffer a stroke than women who walked less than an hour a week.

Diabetes

Moderate activity has been shown to lower the risk of developing diabetes even in women of normal weight. A 16-year study of 68,907 initially healthy female nurses found that those who were sedentary had twice the risk of developing diabetes, and those who were both sedentary and obese had 16 times the risk when compared with normal-weight women who were active.

Remember the study we mentioned above that randomly assigned 3,234 pre-diabetic men and women to modest physical activity (at least 150 minutes a week)? It found exercise to be more effective than the drug Metformin at preventing full-blown diabetes.

Dementia

As the population continues to age, perhaps the greatest health benefit of regular physical activity will turn out to be its ability to prevent or delay the loss of cognitive functions. A study of 3,485 healthy men and women older than 55 found that those who were physically active, three or more times a week, were least likely to become cognitively impaired.

One study conducted in Australia and published in September 2008 in The Journal of the American Medical Association randomly assigned 170 volunteers who reported memory problems to a six-month program of physical activity or health education. A year and a half later, the exercise group showed "a modest improvement in cognition." Various other studies have confirmed the value of exercise in helping older people maintain useful short-term memory, enabling them to plan, schedule, multitask, store information, and use it effectively.

Dr. Carm's Recipe for Staying Active:

- Move every day.

- Optimally, exercise 45 minutes a day, most days of the week.

- Exercise enough to get your heart pounding.

- Do something you love (even if it's cleaning the house).

One thing my mother taught me was that there are many types of exercise. Walk: it is cheap (you just need a pair of sneakers), readily available (outside or in a mall) and can give you time to listen to some music or have some peaceful meditation. Of course, do check with your doctor before you undertake any exercise regimen.

Oh, and don't forget, wipe your dog's ass with ammonia and he might outlive you!

5

The Power of Sleep
or
"After all, even if she's dead, we'll have to wait for the spring thaw to bury her."

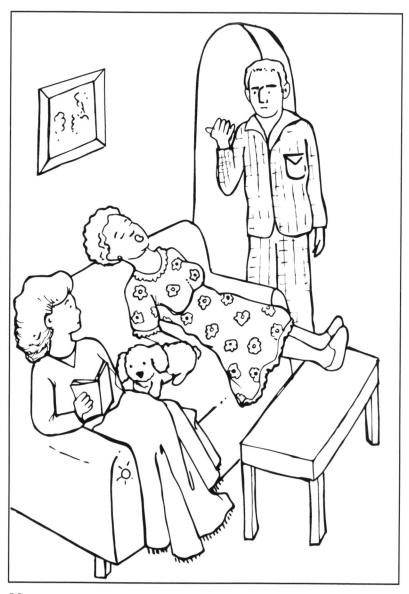

In my family, we believe in sleep. In addition to a full eight hours each night, my mom and dad were both "nappers." I remember one cold winter when, as usual, mom feel asleep while watching television. Dad came in from another room and told me to not disturb her. "Cover her with a blanket; because even if she's dead, we will have to wait for the spring thaw to bury her."

Researchers have shown that sleep improves learning, memory and creative thinking.

No one can argue that a lack of sleep is a real problem today in America. I've seen estimates that 50 to 70 million adults in the United States suffer from a sleeping or wakefulness disorder.

Consider this:

- Every year, there are at least 1,500 deaths as a result of fatigued, drowsy and sleepy drivers.

- There are at least 40,000 injuries reported every year, caused by sleepy drivers.

- Approximately 62 percent of American adults have reported driving while sleepy and drowsy.

- Around 37 percent of people have claimed to have dozed off, at least once, while driving.

In addition to causing accidents and injuries, a lack of sleep is increasingly seen as an important health factor. People who are sleep-deprived often have chronic illnesses such as depression, diabetes, obesity and hypertension. People are also at risk for developing certain cancers.

Here are some sleep-related illnesses:

Insomnia is characterized by an inability to initiate or maintain sleep. It may also take the form of early morning awakening (the individual awakens several hours early and is unable to resume sleeping). Difficulty initiating or maintaining sleep may often manifest itself as excessive daytime sleepiness, which characteristically results in functional impairment throughout the day. Before arriving at a diagnosis of primary insomnia, the healthcare provider will rule out other potential causes, such as other sleep disorders, side effects of medications, substance abuse, depression and previously undetected illnesses.

Narcolepsy is the combination of excessive daytime sleepiness (including episodes of irresistible sleepiness) combined with sudden muscle weakness. The sudden muscle weakness seen in narcolepsy may be elicited by strong emotion or surprise. Episodes of narcolepsy have been described as "sleep attacks" and may occur in unusual circumstances, such as walking and other forms of physical activity. The healthcare provider may treat narcolepsy with stimulant medications combined with behavioral interventions, such as regularly scheduled naps, to minimize the potential disruptiveness of narcolepsy on the individual's life.

Restless Legs Syndrome (RLS) is characterized by an unpleasant "creeping" sensation, often feeling like it is originating in the lower legs, but often associated with aches and pains throughout the legs. This often causes difficulty initiating sleep and is relieved by movement of the leg, such as walking or kicking. Abnormalities in the neurotransmitter dopamine have often been associated with RLS. Healthcare providers often prescribe a medication to help correct the underlying dopamine abnormality along with a drug to promote sleep continuity in the treatment of RLS.

Snoring may be more than just an annoying habit – it may be a sign of sleep apnea. Persons with sleep apnea characteristically make periodic gasping or "snorting" noises, during which their sleep is momentarily interrupted. Those with sleep apnea may also experience excessive daytime sleepiness, as their sleep is commonly interrupted and may not feel restorative. Treatment of sleep apnea is dependent upon its cause. If other medical problems are present, such as congestive heart failure or nasal obstruction, sleep apnea may resolve with treatment of these conditions. Gentle air pressure administered during sleep (typically in the form of a nasal continuous positive airway pressure device) may also be effective in the treatment of sleep apnea. As interruption of regular breathing, or obstruction of the airway during sleep, can pose serious health complications, symptoms of sleep apnea should be taken seriously. Treatment should be sought from a healthcare provider.

Insufficient sleep has been linked to the development of a number of chronic diseases and conditions, including diabetes, cardiovascular disease, obesity, and depression. Research has found that insufficient sleep is linked to an increased risk for the development of type 2 diabetes. Specifically, sleep duration and quality have emerged as predictors of levels of Hemoglobin A1c, an important marker of blood sugar control. Several research articles suggest that optimizing sleep duration and quality may be an important means of improving blood sugar control in persons with type 2 diabetes.

Laboratory research has found that short sleep duration results in metabolic changes that may be linked to obesity. Epidemiological studies have also revealed an association between short sleep duration and excess body weight. This association has been reported in all age groups – but has been particularly pronounced in children. It is believed that sleep in childhood and adolescence is particularly important for brain development and that insufficient sleep in youngsters may adversely affect the function of a region of the brain known as the hypothalamus, which regulates appetite and energy levels.

How much sleep do you need?

Sleep guidelines from the National Sleep Foundation below show how the need for sleep changes as we age:

NEWBORNS (0–2 months)
12–18 hours

INFANTS (3–11 months)
14–15 hours

TODDLERS (1–3 years)
12–14 hours

PRESCHOOLERS (3–5 years)
11–13 hours

SCHOOL-AGE (5–10 years)
10–11 hours

TEENS (10–17 years)
8.5–9.25 hours

ADULTS
7–9 hours

(Taken from the National Sleep Foundation's website.)

The prior sleep requirements include naps. In 2009, the Harvard Health Letter reported that a daytime nap can be good for you. For years, we believed that a daytime nap would interfere with a good night's sleep. New research is showing that a daytime snooze may have health benefits without interfering with nighttime sleep. And while some people worry about napping more as they get older, new research suggests that adding daytime sleep to your schedule can make up for the normal, age-related decay in the quality of nighttime sleep.

Dr. Carm's Recipe for a Restful Sleep:

In accordance with the National Sleep Foundation recommendations:

- Go to bed at the same time each night and rise at the same time each morning.

- Make sure your bedroom is a quiet, dark and relaxing environment – neither too hot nor too cold.

- Make sure your bed is comfortable and use it only for sleeping and not for other activities, such as reading, watching TV, or listening to music. Remove all TVs, computers, and other "gadgets" from the bedroom.

- Physical activity may help promote sleep, but don't do it within a few hours of bedtime.

- Avoid large meals before bedtime.

In addition:

- If your sleep problems persist, or if they interfere with how you feel or function during the day, you should seek evaluation and treatment by a physician.

- Keep a diary of your sleep habits for about ten days to discuss at the doctor's visit.

- Note when you sleep, how much caffeine you drink, and how much alcohol you consume.

The Harvard Health Letter offers some tips for napping:

- Keep it short. A 20- to 30-minute nap may be ideal. Even just napping for a few minutes has benefits. Longer naps can lead to grogginess.

- Find a dark, quiet, cool place. Reducing light and noise helps most people get to sleep faster. Cool temperatures are helpful, too.

- Plan on it. Waiting until sleepiness gets so bad that you have to take a nap can be dangerous if you're driving. A regular nap time may also help you get to sleep faster and wake up quicker.

- Don't feel guilty! A nap can make you more productive at work and at home.

6

Nurture Good Relationships
or
"I'd kill him, but I'd get the chair."

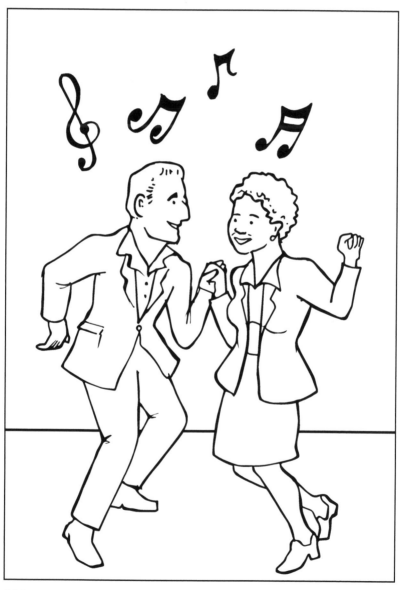

It was no surprise that Mom and Dad passed away within 13 months of each other. They basically did everything together all the years that they knew one another.

I remember many times when my mother and father used to have a "blow out." A "blow out" is a fight involving screaming, cursing and someone (usually Dad) storming out of the house promising never to return. The first few times, I really thought he would not return. It took me a year or two to realize that he was always coming back. It's like he couldn't stay away. Even when my mother would do something that might have caused many men to leave for good, he came back.

And she was no different. More than once we heard her say, "I'd kill him, but I'd get the chair."

Truth was she couldn't last even 13 months without him.

My parents knew that marriage was work, and

they were hard workers. It's now, years later, that I realize that this work, maintaining their relationship, probably extended their lives by years.

Studies suggest that whom you live with – and whether you're single, married, divorced or widowed – can offer clues to your health decades later. Sociologist Linda Waite of the University of Chicago published her research five years ago in her book *The Case for Marriage: Why Married People Are Happier, Healthier, and Better Off Financially*. Divorces and widowhood create stress, which is associated with chronic health problems, she says. And studies show this stress can also have repercussions years later.

Couples who live alone – or with their own children – had equal health advantages. Those in a happy remarriage had better health than the still-divorced or widowed, but not as good as those remaining in one-time marriages. On some physical health measures, they still had a "scar" of divorce or widowhood years later, Waite said.

She then re-analyzed data from more than 8,600 people, ages 51 to 61, to look deeper into their physical and mental health as well as physiological functioning. She says marriage's benefits derive from social connection, risk sharing, specialization of household tasks, and economies of scale.

There is also research into the benefits of emotional connections with people other than spouses or significant others. John Cacioppo, a neuroscientist at the University of Chicago and coauthor of a new book, *Loneliness: Human Nature and the Need for Social Connection*, talked with *U.S. News & World Report* about the latest research on how relationships affect physical health.

"When all is said and done, [one of] the best guarantee[s] of a long and healthy life may be the connections you have with other people." He continues, "This makes sense if you think about early human history. Our... survival required the protection of families and tribes so isolation meant death. The painful feeling known as loneliness is a prompt to reconnect to others."

How does loneliness link to bad health outcomes?

According to Cacioppo, "Loneliness shows up in measurements of stress hormones, immune function, and cardiovascular function. Lonely adults consume more alcohol and get less exercise than those who are not lonely. Their diet is higher in fat, their sleep is less efficient, and they report more daytime fatigue. Loneliness also disrupts the regulation of cellular processes deep within the body, predisposing us to premature aging."

In humans, perceived isolation is so much more important than physical isolation. So, feeling isolated is just as damaging to your health as actually being isolated is.

"Just like hunger and thirst and pain, loneliness signals something important for the survival of your genes – the need for connection to other individuals," Cacioppo says. "A loneliness response might tell you to pass up that promotion that requires that you rip yourself away from friends and family and move to another country. Or, if you do move, you'll know you have to say, 'OK, I will set up a system to maintain and restore those relationships.'"

Dr. Carm's Recipe for Healthy Relationships:

- Develop and nurture positive relationships. Avoid those people who are negative and suck the energy out of you.

- Work on your marriage. Don't expect

that a good marriage just comes naturally. Anything that is going to last a long time (like a house) requires maintenance and attention.

- Cultivate friendships.

- If you are interested in spirituality, by all means, make that an opportunity to connect. Churchgoers, for example, regularly live longer than non-churchgoers. Religious institutions can be very beneficial.

7

Be Your Own Health Advocate
or
"Trust but verify..."

Maybe healthcare wasn't quite as complex 30 years ago. Nevertheless, Mom was good at working it. She knew how to get what she wanted out of people. That included me. Forget that I was her daughter. Forget that I was a practicing healthcare professional. Forget that my advice was free.

Mom: "Wow, Carmella, you really are smart."

Me: "Oh, well, that's nice of you to say. What makes you say that?"

Mom: "Well, remember what you told me about Uncle Frank and his cancer? I checked with Bobby (the pharmacist) and you were right about that treatment."

Me: "Gee, thanks mom. Glad it helped."

When it came to healthcare, she advocated for not only close family, but also extended family and friends.

What made her so effective?

First, she was not afraid to ask anything. Also, she never doubted that her concerns were important. She was polite to a fault, and she double-checked EVERYTHING. She never took the word of just one person, no matter how respected, credible, or closely related they were.

Medicine is a relationship-based business. Knowing what you want, using a punch list, and saying "thank you" will enable you to manage those relationships and move things forward.

Step #1: Know what you want out of the visit or call.

Make a list before the call or visit and include all of your questions. After all, how many times do we walk out of a meeting, or hang up the phone, and then remember what we really wanted?

Step #2: Do your homework.

You'd never walk into a car dealer and say, "Hey, that's a nice car. I don't know what it is, or anything about it, but what color does it come in?" The same is true for healthcare. You need to educate yourself. WebMD is a great resource. Use it to look up symptoms, side effects, and anything else of concern to you.

Many folks are afraid that they may offend their physician if they bring in research. If that does happen, run – don't walk. A good physician-patient relationship should feel like a partnership. Doctors don't know everything.

With my primary care physician, I bring in statistics, articles, and research all the time. My doctor may go to a conference and hear a few new things. But she may not have read the latest article online. The last time I was there, she noted that I needed a boost in medication and asked me if I wanted to let her know what I thought was appropriate. I said, "Absolutely."

Now, you don't need this same level of involvement in your healthcare. It's up to you. The important thing is that you have a physician who will work with you based on your unique desires. You own your body. Nobody else does.

Step #3: Know your rights.

Don't allow yourself to be bullied. If your doctor

is late, that's understandable. Once. If it happens again, let your feet do the talking. Also, read your healthcare contracts carefully. I've worked for health insurance companies for 20 years and have been involved in member appeals and grievances. You have the right to an advocate appointed by the insurer. You can also ask your physician to write letters to support a claim. Don't be shy.

God knows my mother wasn't.

Step #4: Have your "to-do list" ready before you leave for the doctor's and make sure that when the visit is over, you clearly understand:

- The timing of your next appointment.

- Everything about your prescriptions, including side effects.

- Whether you need any additional testing, and if so, whether you have the right paperwork.

- If you need to see a specialist.

Remember that a pen and paper are your best defense against a faulty memory.

Step #5: When you're getting off the phone with your health insurer, make sure you know:

- To whom you spoke.

- What they promised to do, and by when.

- What you need to send and where you need to send it.

Jot down phone numbers and addresses to make following-up easier.

Give thanks.

Of course, no relationship is perfect, but if you appreciate your physician, by all means, say so! When I see my doctor, I not only bring in questions, lists of medications, and articles off the Internet – I also bring a little gift once or twice a year. Because anyone who can deal with me deserves a treat!

Advocating for Parents

When I was in residency in the late 1980s, I discovered that being dead on a ventilator is not the way to go. I saw families torn apart by decision making for a loved one. So I initiated a conversation with Mom and Dad and asked them what they wanted.

Dad was clear. He did not want any extraordinary measures. Mom, on the other hand, said she wanted everything. Furthermore, she urged me not to make her MY healthcare advocate because "no matter what you want, I could never pull the plug on you."

Here are some things you need to think about so that you – and no one but you – decides how you will die.

First: Know yourself.

Be honest about your current state of health.

Know how you want to spend your last days on earth.

Make your wishes very clear to your loved ones. If it's not written, it won't be done.

Second: Get a good lawyer.

There is a whole legal specialty that deals with Elder Law, end-of-life issues, and healthcare advocacy. Get one and take their advice. It's worth a couple hundred dollars to have peace of mind.

Third: Choose an advocate.

Remember that over 50percent of marriages end in divorce. So, as opposed to immediately giving your spouse this responsibility, ask yourself:

Who shares my values?

Who knows my healthcare history?

Who has the means to "advocate" for me? This includes the time and money to be there for you when you need them.

Here are 10 signs that your significant other should NOT be your healthcare advocate:

#10: When your S.O. sees a picture of Brangelina, he/she foams at the mouth and makes embarrassing noises.

#9: When you were in labor, your S.O. wanted to be there but had a "deadline."

#8: He/she refers to you as having the physique of

a "linebacker." Yes, I knew someone who said that to his wife in a room full of people!

#7: He/she has a Swiss bank account, which is news to you.

#6: He/she plans for the future and then asks what you'll be doing.

#5: Out of the 9,000 diapers that your children have soiled, your significant other has not changed one.

#4: He/she thinks that multi-tasking is chewing and swallowing at the same time.

#3: He/she genuflects in the presence of medical professionals.

#2: He/she thinks that "cardiology" is an advanced study of card playing.

#1: Your S.O. never holds back your hair while you throw up.

Qualities of a good advocate:

Your advocate should be geographically close,

have the ability to leave a job when you need him or her, and be competent enough to handle the responsibility. Have an alternate in case your first choice cannot fulfill his or her duties.

Let me tell you why my husband is the guy to pull my plug when the time is right. Mom called me at the office one day and was very upset. She couldn't find her dentures. She had a routine of cleaning them every night in a Styrofoam cup near the bathroom sink. Please don't ask me why. Anyway, she was beside herself because she was sure that she threw them out. And the garbage bags were on the street waiting for the garbage men to pick them up.

Me: "Well, just go outside and get the bags and see if they're in there."

Mom: "I can't. I'm too nervous. Can you come and do it?"

Me: "Mom, I'm at work… "

Just then, Lou called. I merely mentioned what happened, but he immediately left what he was doing, ran over to Mom's, and searched three garbage bags until he found them.

Dr. Carm's Recipe for Healthcare Advocacy:

• Know what you want, be honest about your health and mortality, and be honest about your relationships.

• Get good professional help.

• Document everything and share the documents with family and friends.

• Get an advocate who you trust and who respects your wishes.

• Start this process early and update your documents every three to five years. Life will change, and your documents will need to reflect those changes and reflect your desires accurately.

• Pick an advocate that would fish your mom's teeth out of the bottom of a garbage bag.

8

The Importance of Sex
or
"IT was big. And IT was hard…"

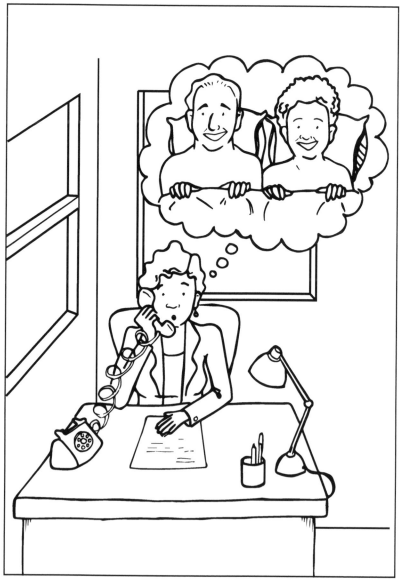

It was a day I'll never forget. I was working for Blue Cross of Northeastern Pennsylvania and the phone rang. It was Mom.

She usually called me several times a day. Most of the time I was in a meeting or doing work. But that was fine with her, because she'd just talk to my assistant, Kelly.

This time, however, she caught me at my desk.

We started with small talk. I was looking out the window and wondering if the sky would ever have sunshine again. It was so gray. No white, no yellow, just gray.

Mom: "Your dad is driving me nuts."

That was not an unusual comment, so I wasn't expecting much.

Me: "Why?"

119

Mom: "Well, you know, he won't leave me alone."

Me: "What do you mean?"

Mom: "You know, he wants to fool around."

Now, at this point, I saw three options …

"Oh, Mom, my boss just walked in, gotta go."

"Oh God, Mom, I really don't want to talk about this!"

"Well, Mom, why is that bothering you?"

Now, I should mention that they were in their late 70s and early 80s at the time. The visual was like a painful, blinding light. I had to blink a couple of times and shake my head.

Me: "Well, Mom, why is that bothering you?"

Mom: "Well, he just won't let me get my cleaning done and I have to make supper."

Me: "Well, you know, a lot of women would be happy. He obviously still finds you attractive after all of these years."

Mom: "Well, sure. I still got it. He goes crazy when I wear that sweater that John and Josette got me for Christmas."

Again, the light!

Me: "And this means that dad is in pretty good health."

Mom: "Why?"

Me: "Well, many men as they age have issues with potency."

Mom: "With what?"

Me: "You know, they can't get an erection."

Mom: "Oh, your father is VERY healthy. Let me tell you. IT was big. And IT was hard."

Me: "Oh, Mom, my boss just walked in. Gotta go!" The light!!

A recent study by the Western Australian Centre for Health and Aging, involving 2,783 Australian men between the ages of 75 and 95 revealed that not only are elderly men still getting it on, but many also wish they were having even more sex. Of the men surveyed, nearly one-third reported having intercourse at least once in the previous year, including 11 percent of men over 90. Among these sexually active men, 43 percent reported not getting as much sex as they would like.

Predictably, "younger" men were more sexually active than older men. Forty percent of the 75- to 79-year-olds reported enjoying an active sex life. Among those who weren't having sex, nearly 50 percent cited physical limitations, such as prostate-related illnesses, and 41 percent reported a lack of interest. Other reasons for a slowdown included low testosterone levels, side effects from medications, and a spouse's lack of interest or physical limitations.

For men, there are several key effects of aging on sexual health:

Testosterone plays a critical role in a man's sexual experience. Testosterone levels peak in the late teens and then gradually decline. Most men notice a difference in their sexual response by age 60 to 65.

The penis may take longer to become erect, and erections may not be as firm. (That is what I was trying to tell Mom... I should have just said, "Dad, you da man!")

It may take longer to achieve full arousal and to have orgasmic and ejaculatory experiences. Erectile dysfunction also becomes more common. Several medications are available to help men achieve and sustain adequate erections.

Let me say this about women, aging and sex: menopause sucks! I have had EVERY symptom documented in the books within the last several years. Some I have actually enjoyed, like the fact that I just don't give a damn what anyone thinks of me anymore. What freedom!

However, the night sweats are no fun. The big boobs that don't fit into shirts are no fun. The weight gain sucks. Period. What about the vaginal dryness and itching? Well, let's just say that I bought stock in the company that makes Astroglide. Astroglide is a vaginal lubricant. Be forewarned about that stuff: it is very powerful. The first time my husband and I used it, we applied too much and with the first thrust, the poor man flew off the bed and almost knocked himself out.

Talk about liftoff!

As women approach menopause, their estrogen levels decrease, which may lead to vaginal dryness and slower sexual arousal. Can you say Mojave Desert? Women may experience emotional changes as well. (Does attacking a man in the supermarket for allegedly stealing your cart count?)

One surprising development is the growth of STDs (sexually transmitted diseases) among our seniors. With the combination of Viagra and Internet dating, seniors now have the ability and the opportunity to have more sex. With this, of course, comes the possibility of sexually transmitted diseases. According to the AARP's 2009 "Sex, Romance and Relationships Survey," of 1,670 men and women:

Five percent of men and women were diagnosed with human papillomavirus, including genital warts.

Seven percent of men, and two percent of women, were diagnosed with gonorrhea.

Three percent of men and women had herpes.

One percent had HIV/AIDS.

One percent had syphilis.

Cases of chlamydia and gonorrhea are on the upswing for those 45 years and older. Chlamydia rates jumped from 361 cases in 2002 to 527 in 2007. Gonorrhea increased from 549 in 2002 to 686 in 2007.

People of all ages should know how to practice safe sex. If you're having sex with a new or different partner, always use a condom. Also talk with your doctor about other ways to protect yourself from sexually transmitted infections.

If you're in a long-term monogamous relationship and you've both tested negative for sexually transmitted infections, you probably don't need to worry about protection. Until you know for sure, however, use a condom when you have sex.

While some women may enjoy sex later in life because they don't have to worry about pregnancy, naturally occurring changes in body shape and size may cause others to feel less sexually desirable. My mom never had this last problem as far as I could tell. She was an innately confident person. She had me when she was 40. So, if we do the math, she was 49 at the time of the following story.

I was in fourth grade and went to a school (The Garfield) with an outside playground that you had to walk through to get into the building. So at 49 years of age, mom would drop me off late to school. (This happened a lot; material for another book...) And she'd drive up in full view of the entire playground.

One day, the resident bully, Sammy, started screaming as I was getting out of the car.

Sammy: "Carmella's mom is naked!"

Now everyone turns to stare and Sammy is beyond excited, waving his little arms with wide eyes like I'd never seen before or since. He was probably experiencing his first little hard-on.

Sammy: "She is in the car and doesn't have a top on."

Well, of course she had a top on.

A tube top!

The woman with the 40D bosom, at the age of 49, was sporting a white terrycloth tube top!

Just imagine what guts it would take to do that.

When I went home that night and reported Sammy's outburst and my mortification, she and my father just laughed.

Years later, she was driving me and some friends to high school one morning, and ran a stop sign. We got pulled over by the police.

Mom: "Oh, officer, I'm so sorry. As you can see I was rushing around and was so afraid that I was going to get them to school late that I didn't even have time to change into clothes."

Yes, she was wearing her nightgown. And yes, he let her go.

There is no doubt in my mind that this self-confidence and self-love was critical for attracting my dad and then "keeping" him for 51 years.

Mom was excellent about transferring that confidence to me. Even when I was an obese pre-teen with acne, a hooked nose and failing grades in astronomy, I remember her telling me that I was a "beautiful, intelligent, funny and amazing person." She said it so many times, and with such enthusiasm, that I actually believed her.

I remember when I realized that my sense of self was not typical among my female teenage friends. Rose, my best friend since we were two years old, frequently had both boys and girls stop over at her house on Pine Street for impromptu get-togethers. Nothing fancy, just pizza, TV, and records (the vinyl kind).

One day she called and asked me to come down as a couple of girls and a couple of boys (all friends of ours) were coming over. I went. We had a good time. Everyone left and I was still there.

I was sitting in the rocker in the living room and Rose pulled up a chair and got really close. She leaned in and asked a question with a very serious tone.

She said, "I don't understand something."

Me: "What?"

Rose: "Well, I spent 40 minutes getting ready and still don't feel like I look my best. But you come walking in with a pair of sweatpants and a red tube top (of course!), no hair done, and no makeup."

Me: "Yeah?"

Rose: "Well, you think you look great, don't you?"

Me: "Yeah."

Rose: "How is that possible?"

I'm not sure what I answered. But it was years later in one of my first jobs when my CEO told me I was an "average" medical director that I realized that I NEVER felt average. I think that if someone who loves you tells you consistently that you are "beautiful, intelligent and amazing," even you will believe it.

Dr. Carm's Recipe for a Healthy Sex Life:

- Sex is a natural and pleasurable part of a healthy relationship. It is another way to communicate. Enjoy it for life.

- Be willing to talk about what you like and what you don't like.

- Use protection. Remember the public service announcement from the 1970s: "VD is for everybody, not just for the few."

- "You are beautiful and intelligent, funny, and an amazing person." If you do not truly believe this, work on this first and then work on the sex. The best sex is when you feel great about yourself. Yes, sometimes we have to "fake" the confidence a bit. Everyone does at one time or another.

- Tell the people you love that they are "beautiful and intelligent, funny, and amazing people," and they will eventually believe it.

- Wear tube tops...

9

The Sandwich Generation
or
"Mental fatigue will kill ya."

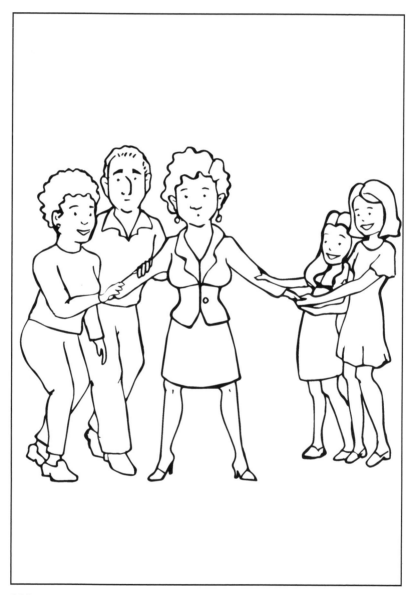

M om never said, "I'm stressed." Her term for stress was "mental fatigue," which I think is beautiful because it is so descriptive. Recently, after a particularly grueling week at work, I thought, "Wow, I'm mentally fatigued. So this is what she meant." I was so tired of thinking that I literally had to lie down.

Stress generated from competing priorities and multitasking will suck the energy right out of you. What gets us to the point of exhaustion is different for everyone.

Let's look at some of the common stressors and what you can do about them.

The Sandwich Generation

They call us the "Sandwich Generation" and for good reason. You feel like a piece of salami "sandwiched" between your children who are still dependent upon you and your parents who are trying like hell not to be.

This concept wasn't in existence in mom's day for a couple of reasons. First, parents didn't live long enough to be one slice of bread, and second, women had children earlier so the responsibilities didn't collide.

My dad's health began to fail first. He struggled to retain the ability to drive. But when that was gone, he lost hope. He stayed at home until he couldn't manage any longer. About a month before he passed, he went to inpatient hospice.

Mom was very upset with me for suggesting hospice, but dad LOVED it. He got so much attention with his sharp wit. While getting a sponge bath one day, he ended up at eye level with the large breasts of one of the nurses and said, "Oh my God, I've died and I'm in heaven!" He told me that his time in hospice was among his most peaceful ever.

Mom fought to hide her illness from me. She was in Pennsylvania and I was in Florida. She knew that if I thought there was anything wrong, I'd make her move. She didn't want that. Running a home is a big thing for most of us. And it can be even more important as we age, since that might be all we have left.

Mom came down for a visit on Dec. 8, 2008 and had a mild heart attack on the 16th. She was recovering in the hospital when I told her that I'd gotten her an apartment in Florida. Within a minute, her heart stopped and she promptly died. She was gone on December 20th, 13 months after my father.

Now, I'm starting to navigate the empty nest. My oldest daughter is a freshman at college and my younger one will soon be as well. On the one hand, you feel so proud. But you also worry about them. And you empathize. It's such an emotional time for everyone. But it's up to you to hold it together.

After we dropped my daughter off at school for the first time, I focused on getting back into my routine. We all thrive on routines and mine begins with a morning workout. When you get your heart pumping and work up a sweat, you literally clear away stressful lines of thinking, increase endorphins, and relieve your body of stress hormones like cortisol. So you navigate life a lot better.

A sweaty workout followed by a deep-tissue massage will give you a healthy glow for days, which is also a great mood booster. Just make sure you drink a lot of water.

The bottom line is that you MUST take care of yourself before you can care for anyone else. We all know this intuitively but still have difficulty putting it into practice. Make a routine of good healthy habits. Write them on your calendar, if you must. Follow them 80percent of the time and you will be a better mother or father and son or daughter.

The toxicity of the electronic-virtual world.

Work-wise, I spend most of my time on the road now giving speeches and presentations. Let's just say, traveling is not what it once was. These days, I dread everything, from strip-search security to bedbug checks.

On top of the travel, we are bombarded by electronic communications. What once could be said in a five-minute phone call is now 10 emails that I have to read while joining a meeting that is taking place in the stratosphere.

It is all a bit much.

The worst part of the travel and the electronics is the perceived lack of control. Nothing can generate stress in your life thinking that you have absolutely no say over what will happen next. I'm a Type A personality, and that focus has been good to me, but at this time in my life, I've had to let go. This acceptance has done more for my overall health than almost anything else.

Here is how to let go:

First, dump the toxicity. I do what makes me feel good. It has taken me a while to find out what works for me. Give yourself time and explore different avenues. For me, taking time to be alone with my thoughts and honoring whatever comes up in the process is very helpful. That may require a spa day, meditation, or vigorous exercise to really get my thoughts flowing. I get some of my best ideas on the spin bike during a class.

In addition, I really have no time or energy for toxic people any longer. I'm not talking about people who need my help. I always have time for that. I am talking about those people who do not have your best interests at heart. Deep down you know who they are. The more time you spend with them – trying to fix them and their drama – the more mental fatigue you will have and the less time you will have for those people in your life who are nurturing and care about YOU. Surround yourself with people of like-mind and attitude.

Meditation is another great way to dump toxicity. Oprah Winfrey is doing some great interviews on the power of meditation for her new network, OWN, and you can download some full episodes on OWN's website for free as well as find her on cable.

Some of her experts go pretty deep by teaching you how to clear out mental cobwebs entirely. You'd be surprised to discover how many present-day circumstances are based upon past thought patterns. You'll find the exercise worthwhile when you begin to make conscious choices and fill your life with joy and meaning.

Junk in, junk out.

Mom firmly believed that what you did to your insides showed up on your face. But, let's face it – pardon the pun – when you've got a full plate with plenty of work and family responsibilities, the last thing you think about is looking your best. But the funny thing is that when I look good, I feel better.

There are some easy steps that you can take to look good anytime.

For your skin, exfoliation is so important. I've recently discovered the Clarisonic. It's a handheld, electronic brush that does for your skin what Sonicare does for your teeth. It whisks away the top layer of dead skin and gives you a fresh, healthy glow. You use it twice a day for a minute at a time. No fuss, no muss, and it's fantastic for all age groups, including my teenage girls.

When you've consumed lots and lots of water, you may find that the delicate skin on the surface of your face begins to naturally exfoliate a lot faster. That's great news. Speeding up the renewal of those skin cells is a key way that we stay looking young and healthy. Drinking 60-plus ounces of water on a daily basis can be a real chore, but it pays off.

Korean women, known for their beautiful skin, have cultivated the art of exfoliation. Many use saunas and steam rooms to open up their pores and use special exfoliation cloths to then gently scrub their top layer of skin. It takes a little practice, though, and you generally find the cloths mainly in specialty shops. However, Amazon.com has a selection. Look around.

Diet has a major impact on your skin. Regularly eating fruits and vegetables – and drinking smoothies, composed of fruits and vegetables – will set you up for a good, healthy glow. It will also make your nails grow quickly, and fill you up so that you don't reach for foods that tax the body – like fast food, junk food, refined carbs, and too much meat.

In pre-historic days, many of us ate a bag's worth of roughage every day. Meat was a treat. For many of us, that remains a good meal plan.

I've seen Organic Girl's Super Greens at Whole Foods and Publix. They taste great and seem to pack a nutritional punch. Try filling 2/3 of a standard blender with them and add a banana, 1 1/2 cups of blueberries, a couple cups of soy milk or almond milk and a handful of blackberries, raspberries, or strawberries. It's delicious.

We've also talked about exercise. Ever notice how much better your complexion looks when you've just had a sweaty workout? Blood flow to the skin is important for rejuvenation.

Just as effective and a whole lot more enjoyable: sex. A powerhouse of stress relief, increased blood flow, and mighty endorphins!

Too Many priorities.

Managing the work-life balance is another key to stress reduction. When I was in my 30s, I worked for Blue Cross in Pennsylvania, did clinical work on the weekends, was pursuing a master's degree, and had two young children. Fortunately, my husband proved to be a great partner. But I would be lying if I said that we thrived as a family during this time. We survived and that was about it.

As a result of that, I discovered four activities that helped me master my time and schedule. First was learning to prioritize. You have to accept that you cannot have it all. There, I said it. You can have all of it, but not all at the same time. Decide what your priority is for today and then accept that the rest of it will have to wait.

I learned my lesson in prioritizing from... a MAN! Bill was an executive I worked with years ago, who was comfortable in his own skin. Even when under tremendous pressure and while raising five children, he always seemed cool and calm.

How did he do it?

"Some days I go home and I think I did really well

at work today," he told me. "Other days, I am happy with the way I've handled a crisis with my kids or supported my wife. These two things don't happen at the same time. But at the end of the week, if I can look in the mirror and be happy with myself overall, then I did ok."

Prioritizing is one of the most difficult decisions you have to make. But it will pay you back a thousand-fold. If your child has a volleyball game tonight and you are staring at an unfinished report that is due tomorrow, you MUST decide what you will do now and what can wait. Don't think that you can do them both at the same time.

Something that has helped me in this regard is learning to limit my activities so that I can be "present" and focus on one thing at a time.
Second is taking advantage of flexibility – and being flexible. Companies are providing more flexibility than ever, and even though I bitch about electronics and the virtual world, they have allowed me to optimize my time. However, don't forget the fact that YOU must be flexible. Don't think that you are going to change the time of the kid's baseball game, because you aren't, and if the boss expects the report on her desk tomorrow morning at 9 a.m., then it's 9 a.m. Accept this and

adjust your schedule. If the game starts at 6 p.m., work until 5:30, stay at the game until 7:30, and then hustle home and finish that report. That may mean working through the night, but you may decide it's worth it.

Third is planning. This is a critical and non-negotiable tactic to master. It involves both short-term planning (via your calendar) and long-term life planning. In essence you must first prioritize and then take advantage of the external and internal flexibilities that exist in your current life. Then plan. Make lists. Have goals.

Last and certainly not least is setting boundaries. This is something that we women have a whole lot more trouble with than our male counterparts. This involves saying NO. If you are not able to say NO, you are in trouble. You don't have to be mean about it. You can say it with a sweet Southern accent, but it MUST be said.

When it all comes together, here is what it looks like: I, Dr. Carm, have two competing priorities today, my daughter's basketball game and a meeting that will take me to Fort Lauderdale all day. My first priority is getting to see my daughter play her game. I have some flexibility because there are a ton of flights in and out of Tampa and my employer allows me to make my own travel arrangements. I will fly out in the early morning (which requires me to wake up at 4 a.m.) and fly home by 3:30 p.m. This will allow the security people to frisk me (which I sometimes enjoy) and get me home in time to make it to the game. That is my plan.

At some point, I will either get a call that I need to bake brownies and bring them to the game or I will have a call for work at 4:30 p.m. This is where boundaries come in. I buy the damn brownies instead of baking them and I take the call tomorrow unless someone is dying because I have learned to say NO.

Please don't think for a moment that any of this will feel good at the time. You will do this a hundred times and will still feel some guilt. But in the end, you will spend time on what really matters to you and with the people who really matter to you.

So the tools are out there. Just remember to take care of YOU, avoid toxic people, and give up the fallacy of control and "having it all."

Dr. Carm's Recipe for Surviving Mental Fatigue: For Your Parents:

- Ask your parents in advance about their wishes; have "The Talk."

- Find out what they want, and have them sign a power of attorney and a healthcare delegate statement.

- You can easily get these documents right off of the Internet for free, but hire a lawyer, if you can. It's worth the money.

- When tackling end-of-life issues, remember to take care of you. I tried to get enough sleep, didn't stop exercising, ate well, and prayed a lot.

- Stay as empathetic as possible. This will be painful because it's a painful time of life. But it is so critical to honor their wishes and not put yours before theirs.

For Your Kids:

- One study I read said that whatever influence you have on your kids is determined by the sixth grade. If they're going to smoke, do drugs, or have early sex, it's ingrained and learned by then. That's not to say that it can't be unlearned. But if there's an issue, it's best to jump on it early.

- No matter how adult they are becoming, they want to know that they have a place at home, a sanctuary where they will always be safe. So whatever you do, don't change their room until they no longer care.

- They'll start to pull away from you when they get into high school. They may get extra mouthy and not pull their weight. Just stick to your guns and call them out on it. ("I know you're leaving soon. You'll miss me and I'll miss you. Meantime, don't make me go ape shit!")

For YOU:

- Spa days, vigorous exercise, and hot yoga are great ways to refocus and stay big picture in a snap.

- Exfoliate, drink lots of water, and eat lots of fruits and veggies.

- Nix the toxic people. Social networks are a great way to read between the lines. If someone is dedicating precious time to photographing their lunch, how much energy do you think they'll have left over for bigger things.... like you?

- Meditate, listen to quality programs, and broadcasts and read (or listen to) quality books that really get you thinking.

- Set priorities, be flexible, plan your time, and respect your boundaries.

10

The Cook Book
or
"Making it stick."

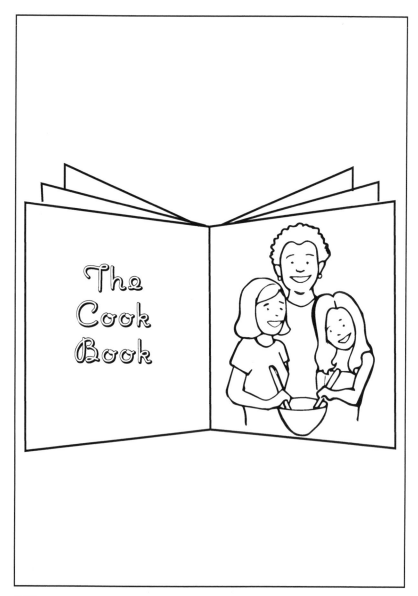

Mom and I did a lot of baking and cooking together. Dad was always there beside her as her sous chef. He would cut up apples for the pie, chop the veggies for soup, and do just about anything she asked of him. Little did I realize at the time that the recipes for the dishes we were cooking up were just a small example of what I was really learning. In this book I've shared stories of our family that teach how all of us can live a healthy and happy life. I've included the empirical medical data that supports the teachings. What I would give today to have my mom and dad beside me as I make a pot of spaghetti sauce, watch my little babies growing into beautiful young women, and marvel at how blessed I am to have married my best friend. I've picked the best of the best from the preceding chapters. I promise that as you incorporate these teachings into your life, you will feel healthy, less stressed, and develop a strange compulsion to wear tube tops. Enjoy!

Dr. Carm's Recipe for Healthy Living:

Ingredients:

- Mostly vegetables and whole fruits and (if you must) a small amount of animal products. If you do eat meat, aim for lean protein. Go easy on all fats and always choose unsaturated; avoid trans fats.

- A "pinch" of dessert. Remember: all things in moderation.

- Almost no fried foods, processed foods, or commercially prepared baked goods (donuts, cookies, crackers).

- Plenty of whole grains. Avoid "white" foods like white flour, bread, pasta, and refined sugar.

- Adequate calcium and Vitamin D.

- Smoking cessation or abstinence.

- Infrequent dining out and copious amounts of sharing when you do.

- Breakfast every day.

- Moderate amounts of alcohol (one drink for women and two max for men per day is the recommendation).

- Move every day. Optimally, get aerobic exercise (walking, biking, etc.) for 150 minutes per week and weight-bearing exercises 40-90 minutes per week. Do something you love; even cleaning the house will do it!

- Adequate sleep. It is critical for a healthy body and mind. Get your seven to eight hours per night and don't be afraid of short naps.

- Cups and cups of positive relationships. Develop, nurture, and work on them. Avoid people who are negative and suck the energy out of you.

- Sex, often. It is a natural and pleasurable part of a healthy relationship. It is another way to communicate. Enjoy it for life.

- Self-confidence. Have it and share it. Tell the people you love that they are "beautiful and intelligent, funny, and amazing people" and they will eventually believe it.

Directions

I have struggled since I was no longer a "skinny baby" with changing my behavior and making the new habits stick. I have learned through success and failure that there are some critical components to any habit change that will ensure that the new behavior becomes automatic.

The components are easy to recall if you can remember my name: DrCARM.

Dr: Destination: Make a plan; have a goal. Make your goal specific, measurable, and timed.

C: Calendar: Schedule your good habit, like exercise, into your day as you would meetings, doctor appointments, etc. This way it will happen.

A: Anticipate: Plan the night before (get clothes ready for gym); plan the week before (make healthy suppers on Sunday and freeze for the week).

R: Record: Journal your thoughts, issues, progress. How did you feel after you exercised? Are you sleeping well?

M: Mate: Get a friend, partner, or pet to encourage you and share the journey to good health. It is best to change one thing at a time.

Incorporate the healthy behavior into your life with the DrCARM tactics and repeat for at least 3 weeks. When you notice yourself performing the new habit without thinking, then the habit is "stuck" and you can move on to the next one.

Please visit me at **www.drcarm.com** and let me know how our recipes work out for you. Oh, and thanks to Mom and Dad.